DATES IN

NEUROLOGY

DATES IN

NEUROLOGY

EDITED BY H.S.J. LEE

The Parthenon Publishing Group
International Publishers in Medicine, Science & Technology

NEW YORK   LONDON

Library of Congress Cataloging-in-Publication Data

Data available on request.

British Library Cataloguing in Publication Data

Dates in neurology. - (Landmarks in medicine series)
    1. Neurology - History - Chronology
    I. Lee, H. S. J.
    616.8′009′0202

    ISBN 1-85070-529-1

Published in the USA by
The Parthenon Publishing Group Inc.
One Blue Hill Plaza
PO Box 1564, Pearl River
New York 10965, USA

Published in the UK and Europe by
The Parthenon Publishing Group Limited
Casterton Hall, Carnforth
Lancs. LA6 2LA, UK

No part of this book may be reproduced in any form without permission from the publishers, except for the quotation of brief passages for the purposes of review.

Printed and bound by Bookcraft (Bath) Ltd., Midsomer Norton, UK

Copyright © 2000 Parthenon Publishing Group

Acknowledgment

The editor would like to acknowledge the National Library of Medicine, World Health Organization and the Nobel Foundation for provision of illustrations.

Introduction

Modern understanding of neurology is based on the achievements and contributions of many doctors and scientists over many years. To appreciate the state-of-the-art as it exists today, it is helpful to know something of the background and history of the subject as it has developed over the last few centuries – and as the underlying scientific principles have become more fully understood and elucidated.

This volume records some of the key milestones in the development of modern neurology that have taken place over the millennium. Of course, although some notable contributions were made in earlier centuries, it is really only in the later years of the present millennium that advances in knowledge and practice become numerous and significant. Naturally, too, these advances are closely related to progress in other fields of medicine – and this fact is also reflected in the pages of the book.

The milestones listed here are indeed important ones but are by no means comprehensive. Readers will all have their own individual views of additional important events that should be recorded, and I would certainly welcome their suggestions for the next edition.

It is hoped that the milestones described will provide an interesting reference and aide-memoire to all those with an interest in neurology who would like to know more about its background and development. At the start of the new millennium it seems appropriate to look back and chart the dramatic progress that has been made in the course of the preceding one.

c. 3000BC Trephination was undertaken in nearly all parts of the world and continued until the Middle Ages.

c. 2820BC SHEN NUNG born.
A Chinese emperor, physician and reformer who originated acupuncture and wrote the great herbal *Pen Tsoa*.

c. 1700BC The Smith Papyrus, an Egyptian medical treatise, was written. It contains the first record of the nervous system.

c. 520BC ALCMAEON OF CROTON, a Greek philosopher and physiologist, dissected animals and studied their brains, and discovered the optic nerve.

460BC HIPPOCRATES born.
A physician in ancient Greece, regarded as the father of medicine, who separated medicine from superstition. His *Corpus Hippocraticum* includes treatments for all medical conditions known at this time.

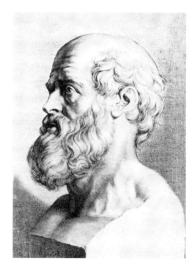

Hippocrates
(460–377)

355BC   HEROPHILUS OF CHALCEDON born.
A Greek physician from Asia Minor who, while working in Alexandria, was the first to recognize the brain as the center of the nervous system and seat of intelligence.

c. 340BC   ERASISTRATUS born.
One of the first anatomists at the Alexandrian school who accurately described complicated structures, such as the convolutions and the ventricles of the brain.

25BC   AULUS CORNELIUS CELSUS born.
A Roman physician who wrote *De Medicina*, a treatise divided into three parts: dietetic, pharmaceutical, and surgical. It contained the first accounts of hydrotherapy, lateral lithotomy, and insanity.

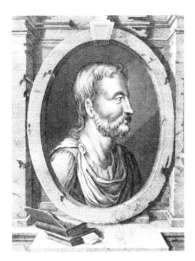

Aulus Cornelius Celsus
(25 BC–AD 50)

98AD   SORANUS OF EPHESUS born.
A Greek physician who practiced in Alexandria and Rome and described nervous disorders and their treatment in *On Acute and Chronic Diseases*.

c. 100   ARETAEUS OF CAPPADOCIA, a physician from Asia Minor, distinguished between spinal and cerebral paralysis, described elephantiasis, and manic depression.

129   CLAUDIUS GALEN born.
The most famous of the Roman physicians who founded the Galenic system of medicine, which was followed for 1500 years until the Renaissance when it was questioned by ANDREAS VESALIUS and PARACELSUS.

625   PAUL OF AEGINA born.
An Alexandrian physician and surgeon, famed for his *Epitomae medicae libri septem*, which included descriptions of trephining and paracentesis, and also dealt with apoplexy and epilepsy.

850   RHAZES born.
An Arab physician, considered the greatest physician of the Islamic world. He wrote many medical texts, among them *Liber Continens*, an encyclopedia of medical practice and treatment, and gave the first description of smallpox and measles.

930   HALY ABBAS born.
An Arab physician whose principal work, *Kamil al-sina'a al-tibbiya* was divided into two sections on theoretical and practical medicine. Each section contained 10 tracts on specialized topics.

965   ALHAZEN born.
An Arab mathematician and physician from Basra who made significant contributions to optical theories. His treatise *Kitab Al-Manazir* included theories on refraction, reflection and the study of lenses, and gave the first accurate account of vision.

980 AVICENNA born.
An Arab physician and philosopher–scientist who wrote a vast scientific and philosophical encyclopedia, *Kitab-ash-shifa* and a treatise on medicine, *al-Quanum fil-Tibb* in five volumes.

1201 WILLIAM OF SALICETO born.
An Italian cleric, physician and surgeon who wrote *Chyrurgia*. He described the suture of severed nerves, and gave one of the earliest accounts of dropsy resulting from a kidney disorder (Bright disease).

1280 Italian physician and philosopher, PETER OF ABANO, proposed the revolutionary idea that the brain was the source of the nerves, and the heart was the source of the blood vessels.

1290 LANFRANC born.
An Italian surgeon from Milan who wrote a system of surgery, *Chirurgia Magna*, and was the first to describe concussion of the brain.

1452 LEONARDO DA VINCI born.
A Renaissance artist, inventor, engineer and anatomist from Italy who accurately produced a wax cast of the ventricles of a human brain.

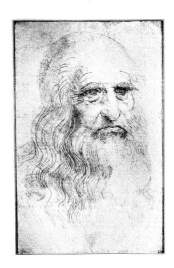

Leonardo da Vinci
(1452–1519)

1470   JACOPO BERENGARIO DA CARPI born.
An Italian anatomist who was noted for his use of
mercurial ointment to treat syphilis. He published *De
fractura calvariae sive cranii* (1518), *Commentaria super anatomia
Mundini* (1521), and *Isagogue* (1522).

1500   VIDIANUS born.
A professor of medicine at Pisa who first described the
nerve of the pterygoid (Vidian nerve) and its artery
(Vidian artery, 1611).

1503   CHARLES ETIENNE born.
A physician from Paris who described the central canal of the
spinal cord. In 1546 he further described morbid cavitation in
the spinal cord (syringomyelia).

1506   JEAN FRANÇOIS FERNEL born.
An eminent French physician who published *Universa Medica*.
He observed that the spinal cord was hollow, and gave a clear
description of the peristaltic action of the alimentary canal.

1515   ANDREAS VESALIUS born.
A Flemish physician who revolutionized the study of
medicine and wrote and illustrated the first comprehensive
textbook of anatomy, *De humani corporis fabrica* (1543), whilst
at the University of Padua.

1520   GUILIO CESARE ARANZI born.
An Italian anatomist who described the choroid plexus,
foramen ovale and ductus arteriosus, and named the
hippocampus of the brain.

1521 CHRISTOPHER LANGTON born.
A London physician who wrote on madness and affections of the mind, and published *An introduction into phisyke, wyth an universal dyet.*

1523 GABRIELE FALLOPPIO born.
An Italian anatomist who discovered the Fallopian tubes of the ovaries, the semicircular canals of the ear, the chorda tympani, and the trigeminal, auditory and glossopharyngeal nerves, described in his *Observationes Anatomicae* of 1561.

1524 BARTOLOMMEO EUSTACHIO born.
A professor of anatomy in Rome who discovered the Eustachian tube, the Eustachian valve in the fetus, the suprarenal bodies and the abducent nerve. He wrote *Opuscula anatomica* published in 1564.

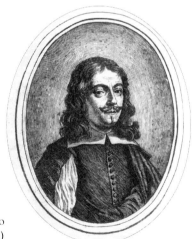

Bartolommeo Eustachio
(1524–1574)

1536 The first book devoted entirely to the anatomy of the head, *Anatomica Capitis Humani*, was written by JOHANNES DRYANDER.

1536 FELIX PLATTER born.
A physician in Basel, Switzerland who was the first to distinguish between various mental disorders. He wrote extensive accounts of psychiatric disorders in his *Praxis Medica* and *Observationum* published in 1602 and 1614, respectively. He described asthma due to obstruction of the small pulmonary arteries or nerve disturbances.

1539 An early account of neurosyphilis was given by an Italian physician from Venice, NICCOLO MASSA.

1543 CONSTANZO VAROLIO born.
An Italian professor of anatomy at Bologna and Rome who described fluid in the brain and the pons (1573), the latter being named pons varoli in his honor.

1549 Vertigo was described as a symptom of brain disease by JASON PRATENSIS, a physician from The Netherlands.

1558 The origin of the optic nerves in the brain was described by Italian anatomist, BARTOLOMMEO EUSTACHIO.

1561 GIULIO CASSERIO born.
An Italian physician and teacher of William Harvey who described the musculocutaneous nerve.

1573 The first clear mention of cerebrospinal fluid (CSF) was made by Italian anatomist, CONSTANZO VAROLIO, of Bologna and Rome.

1592 JACOBUS BONTIUS born.
A physician from Leiden who gave a description of dry beriberi in his *De Medicina Indorum* of 1642.

1596 Arrow poison was mentioned by SIR WALTER RALEIGH in his book *Discovery of the Large, Rich, and Beautiful Empire of Guiana*.

1608 GIOVANNI BORELLI born.
A physiologist and professor of mathematics at Pisa who founded 'Iatrophysics', the use of physical laws to explain bodily functions, and analyzed muscle action and contraction.

1611 The functions of the olfactory nerve were described in Copenhagen, Denmark, by CASPAR BARTHOLIN, THE ELDER.

1621 THOMAS WILLIS born.
An English physician who wrote *Cerebri Anatome, cui accessit Nervorum descriptio et usus* (1664), and *Pathologiae cerebri et nervosi generis specimen* (1667). He is considered the founder of neuroanatomy and neurophysiology.

1622 The involuntary response of the nervous system (reflex action) was described by the French scientist and philosopher, RENÉ DESCARTES, in *Tractatus De Homine*.

1629 EDMUND KING born.
A London physician to Charles II who published an important paper on dissection of the brain in relation to the pineal gland (1686).

1633 WILLIAM CROONE born.
An English physician and anatomist at the Company of Surgeons who suggested that muscle contraction was caused by a reaction to substances passing from nerves.

1637 French scientist and philosopher, RENÉ DESCARTES, published *Dioptrica*, comparing the eye to a camera, and suggesting the nature of reflex reactions.

1641 RAYMOND DE VIEUSSENS born.
A French anatomist who described the anterior medullary velum, central canal of the cochlea columella, and the ansa subclavia of sympathetic nerves, all of which were named after him.

1648 A scientific study of apoplexy, with associated changes in the brain, was published by JOHANN JACOBUS WEPFER, a German physician from Schaffhausen. In 1658 he demonstrated that cerebral hemorrhage was the cause of apoplexy (stroke).

1661 English physician, THOMAS WILLIS, reported on cerebrospinal fever (meningitis).

1663 FRIEDRICH HOFFMANN born.
A German physician who developed the idea that a vital fluid in the nerves gives 'tonus' to the muscles, and wrote *Systema Medicinae Rationalis* and *Medicina Consultoria*.

1663 An early English treatise, *De Morborum Capitis Effentis et Prognosticis*, dealing with cerebral and mental affections and diseases of the head, was published by Englishman, ROBERT BAYFIELD.

1664 *Cerebri Anatome, cui accessit Nervorum descriptio et usus* by THOMAS WILLIS, was published. This contained one of the first descriptions of the brain, the arterial supply to the base of the brain (circle of Willis), and the 11th cranial nerve responsible for motor stimulation of the neck muscles. Willis suggested that the cerebellum controlled involuntary movements, and the cerebrum presided over voluntary movements, and described the aortic depressor nerve, a branch of the vagus supplying the aorta, as a wandering nerve.

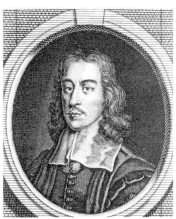

Thomas Willis
(1621–1675)

1665 ANTONIO PACCHIONI born.
An Italian neurologist who studied the structure and function of the dura mater, proposing that it exerted a contractile force on the brain, and described arachnoidal granulations under the dura mater (Pacchioni bodies).

1665 MARCELLO MALPIGHI published *De lingua*, in which he distinguished between the outer layer of the tongue and the reticular mucous layer and isolated the taste buds. His *De cerebro* demonstrated that the white matter of the nervous system was made up of bundles of fibers which connected the brain with the spinal cord.

1667 In his *Pathologiae cerebri et nervosi generis specimen*, THOMAS WILLIS suggested the nervous origins of convulsive disorders such as epilepsy, asthma, apoplexy, narcolepsy, and convulsive coughs. He gave an account of whooping cough, described the role of bronchial innervation, and the late-stage effects of syphilis on the brain.

1668 GIORGIO BAGLIVI born.
A founder of the Iatrophysical School of Medicine in Italy who published *De Praxi Medica* and *Opera Omnia Medico Practica, et Anatomica*, and distinguished between smooth and striped muscle.

1669 JACOB BENIGNUS WINSLOW born.
A Danish anatomist who named the 'grand sympathetic' for the ganglion chain, and called the smaller branches 'lesser sympathetic'.

1671 GEORGE CHEYNE born.
A Scottish physician and eminent writer who wrote *A New Theory of Fevers*, and *The English Malady or Treatise on Nervous Diseases*.

1684 *Neurographia*, was written by French neurologist, RAYMOND DE VIEUSSENS, who also studied white matter of the brain and described the cerebellum, the anterior medullary velum, central canal of the cochlea columella, and ansa subclavia of the sympathetic nerves.

1686 A form of chorea accompanied by involuntary irregular jerky movements in children and young adults (St Vitus dance) was described in *Schedula Monitoria de Nove Febres Ingressu*, by English physician, THOMAS SYDENHAM.

1692 The corpuscles forming small prominences of arachnoid tissue under the dura mater (Pacchioni bodies) were described by Italian professor of anatomy, ANTONIO PACCHIONI.

1694 RICHARD MORTON, physician to James II, described patients suffering from the classic symptoms of anorexia nervosa, calling it nervous atrophy.

1695 The cerebral vessels of the brain were noted by London anatomist and physician, HUMPHREY RIDLEY, in his *The Anatomy of the Brain*, and the coronary sinus (Ridley sinus) is named after him.

1699 One of the first accounts of hydrocephalus was given to the Royal Society by JOHN FRIEND of Northamptonshire.

1706 BENJAMIN FRANKLIN born.
An American scientist and statesman who invented the bifocal lens, pioneered the treatment of nervous diseases using electricity, and wrote on many medical subjects.

1708 ALBRECHT VON HALLER born.
A Swiss anatomist who described several anatomical structures, particularly related to the mechanical automatism of heart muscle function.

1710 WILLIAM CULLEN born.
A Scottish physician who wrote *Synopsis Nosologicae Practicae* (1769) in which he initiated a classification of disease (nosology) into fevers, neuroses, cachexiae and local disorders.

1714 Illustrations from *Tabulae Anatomicae* by Italian anatomist Bartolommeo Eustachio were published by Giovanni Lancisi, 140 years after Eustachio's death. Among them were accurate illustrations of the thoracic duct, facial muscles, the larynx, and the sympathetic nervous system.

1714 Robert Whytt born.
A Scottish professor of medicine who described tuberculous meningitis in children in *Observations on Dropsy of the Brain* (1768), and described hydrocephalus due to the same disease (Whytt disease).

1724 Johann Friedrich Meckel, the Elder born.
A professor of anatomy at Berlin who described the sphenopalatine ganglion (Meckel ganglion) and the dural space (Meckel cavity, 1749) in which the Gasserian ganglion is lodged.

1725 Pierre Tarin born.
A French anatomist who studied the brain and described the thickening of the velum medullare at the vermis of the cerebellum (Tarin valve, 1750).

1731 Allan Burns born.
A Scottish surgeon who wrote *Observations on Some of the Most Important and Frequent Diseases of the Heart* (1809), in which he described phrenic nerve palsy, a sign of thoracic aortic aneurysm, and *Observations on the Surgical Anatomy of the Head and Neck* (1812).

1732 Jacob Benignus Winslow, a Danish anatomist, gave the name 'grand sympathetic' to the ganglion chain and called the smaller branches 'lesser sympathetic'.

1733 ALEXANDER MONRO, SECUNDUS born.
A famous Edinburgh anatomist who published
Observations on the Structure and Function of the Nervous System
(1783), *Three Treatises on the Brain, Eye and
Ear* (1797), and on general anatomy.

1734 JOHANN GOTTLIEB WALTER born.
A professor of anatomy in Berlin who gave his name to the
smallest branch of the splanchnic nerve passing through the
renal plexus.

1736 DOMENICO COTUGNO born.
A professor of anatomy from Naples, Italy, who described
fluid in the brains of fish (1784), several structures of the
labyrinthine apparatus (1760), and gave a classic description
of sciatica.

1737 MICHAEL UNDERWOOD born.
A London pediatrician who gave possibly the first scientific
description of poliomyelitis (1793).

1737 LUIGI GALVANI born.
An Italian physician who wrote one of the first and most
important early texts on electrical stimulation of muscles
(1791).

1739 HEINRICH AUGUST WRIESBERG born.
A German anatomist who described the internal cutaneous
nerve to the minor brachi (named after him).

1741 JOHN JACOB HUBER, a professor of anatomy at Göttingen,
described the aberrant ganglion on the posterior root of the
first cervical nerve.

1742   ANTOINE PORTAL born.
A professor of anatomy at the Jardin du Roi in Paris who
published an important work on epilepsy.

1744   The inferior carotid ganglion in the cavernous plexus
was described by KASIMIR CHRISTOPH SCHMIEDEL, professor
of anatomy and botany at Erlangen.

1745   PHILLIPE PINEL born.
A neuropsychiatrist from Paris who was one of the first
to follow Cullen's psychological theory on insanity, and
to refer to it as an illness, unchain patients, and treat
them humanely, he also recognized dementia as a
separate entity.

1745   PETER JOHANN FRANK born.
A German physician who was the first to focus on diseases of
the spinal cord.

1745   BENJAMIN RUSH born.
An American physician, regarded as the first psychiatrist in
America, who wrote *Diseases of the Mind* (1821), and
introduced occupational therapy in the treatment of mental
diseases.

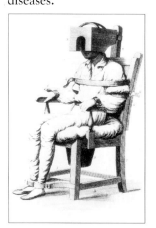

Rush's tranquilizing chair

1745 ALESSANDRO CODIVALLI born.
An Italian surgeon and neurologist who differentiated efferent and afferent nerve action in muscles.

1746 The first monograph on epilepsy, *Cases of Epilepsy, Hysteric Fits, and St Vitus Dance, with the Process of Cure*, was written by JOHN ANDREE, a physician at the London Hospital.

1747 The concept of impulse and irritability of living tissues was introduced in *Primae Lineae Physiologiae* by Swiss physician, ALBRECHT VON HALLER. In 1766 he gave a clear, scientific description of cerebrospinal fluid (CSF).

1749 GEORGIUS PROCHASKA born.
An anatomist at Prague who demonstrated the integrated functions of the brain in producing movements of the body (1779).

1751 Pupillary reaction was established as a reflex reaction in *Essay on Vital and Other Involuntary Motions of Animals*, by Edinburgh neurologist, ROBERT WHYTT. In 1768 he wrote *Observations on Dropsy of the Brain*, and described hydrocephalus due to tuberculose meningitis (Whytt disease).

1752 The first successful operation for a brain abscess (temperosphenoidal abscess following ear infection) was performed by French surgeon, SAUVEUR FRANÇOIS MORAND.

1755 The first use of electroconvulsive therapy for mental illness was by French physician, J B LE ROY.

1758 FRANZ JOSEPH GALL born.
A German physician who gave an early description of the
structure of the brain on a scientific basis, proposed that gray
matter was the active part of the nervous system and that
white matter provided the connections, and established
phrenology.

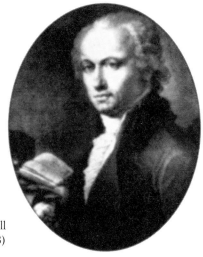

Franz Joseph Gall
(1758–1828)

1759 JOHANN CHRISTIAN REIL born.
A neuroanatomist and physician from Berlin who
described the insula of the cerebral cortex or the lobule
of the corpus striatum, island of Reil (1796), and wrote a
treatise on psychotherapy in 1803.

1761 An identical condition to syncope due to cardiac arrest
or heart block, was described as 'epilepsy with slow pulse'
by the father of Italian anatomy, GIOVANNI BATTISTA
MORGAGNI.

1763 The use of willow in pain relief was suggested and described
by British physician, EDMUND STONE.

1764   A classic description of sciatica was given by DOMENICO COTUGNO, professor of anatomy at Naples, who distinguished two forms: one causing swelling or irritation of the sciatic nerve (Cotugno disease) and the other from inflammation of the hip joint (arthritic sciatica).

1764   JOHN HASLAM born.
A superintendent at the Bethlem Mental Asylum (Bedlam), London who described general paralysis of the insane (1816), examined the brains of the diseased insane at autopsy, and recorded the changes in the brain due to syphilis.

1765   The ganglion of the trigeminal nerve (Gasserian ganglion) was named after Viennese anatomist, JOHANN LAURENTIUS GASSER, by one of his students, ANTON BALTHASAR RAYMOND.

1765   FRANÇOIS RIBES born.
An army surgeon from Toulouse who described the uppermost sympathetic ganglion situated on the anterior communicating artery of the circle of Willis, the ganglion of Ribes (1817).

1767   Nerve generation and the Fontana canal in the eye were noted by Italian anatomist, FELIX F G FONTANA, founder and first director of the Natural History Museum in Florence.

1768   JOSEPH WENZEL born.
A professor of anatomy and physiology from Mainz, Germany who described ventriculus cerebri primus, Wenzel ventricle.

1771 The term 'reflex' was introduced by JOHAN AUGUST UNZER from Halle in Germany to describe the sensory-motor reaction.

1773 LUIGI ROLANDO born.
An anatomist in Turin, Italy, who described the sulcus centralis of the brain (Rolando fissure), studied the cerebellum, and described several other structures of the brain including the Rolandic convolution and Rolandic area.

1773 Trigeminal neuralgia was described by Quaker physician from England, JOHN FOTHERGILL, in *Of a painful affection of the face*, or Fothergill disease. In 1776 he gave a clinical description of migraine headache.

1774 SIR CHARLES BELL born.
A Scottish anatomist, physiologist, and neurologist who recognized that lesions of the 7th nerve could bring about facial palsy (Bell palsy), published *Engravings of the Brain and Nervous System* (1802) and *Idea of a New Anatomy of the Brain* (1811), and explained the part played by the dorsal root in the sympathetic arc reflex (1811).

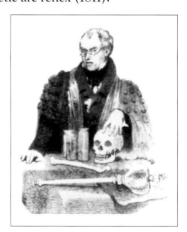

Charles Bell
(1774–1842)

1775 JULIEN JEAN CESAR LEGALLOIS born.
A physician and physiologist from Cherneix in France who proposed the concept of maintaining life without need for the heart, by regular injection or supply of blood, and discovered the respiratory center in the medulla oblongata (1812).

1776 Italian anatomist, FRANCESCO GENNARI, described the laminar structure of the cerebral cortex in the occipital lobe.

1776 CHARLES FREDERICK BURDACH born.
A professor of medicine from Dorpat who described the posterior column of the spinal cord (Burdach column, 1819).

1776 CONRAD JOHANN MARTIN LANGENBECK born.
A surgeon at Göttingen who described the superficial nerve of the scapula (Langenbeck nerve, 1803).

1777 The first clear description of color blindness was given by English physician, JOSEPH HUDDARD, in a letter to JOSEPH PRIESTLEY.

1779 OLAUS ACREL, a Swedish surgeon who pioneered ophthalmic surgery in Scandinavia, described the pseudoganglion on the posterior interosseous nerve at the back of the wrist (Acrel ganglion).

1780 JOHN ABERCROMBIE born.
A surgeon to the Royal Public Dispensary in Edinburgh who wrote *Observations on the Diseases of the Spinal Marrow* (1818) and *Pathological and Practical Researches on Diseases of the Brain and Spinal Cord* (1828), the first book on neuropathology.

1781 FRIEDRICH TIEDEMANN born.
An anatomist at Heidelberg, Germany who described the plexus of nerve fibrils around the central artery of the retina arising from the central ciliary nerves (Tiedemann nerve).

1783 FRANÇOIS MAGENDIE born.
A pioneer of pharmacology and founder of experimental physiology who described the mechanism of deglutition and vomiting (1813), the function of cerebrospinal fluid (1825), and the foramen of Magendie of the brain (1828), a canal leading to the 4th ventricle.

1783 LUDWIG LEVIN JACOBSON born.
An anatomist and physician from Copenhagen who described the tympanic branch of the glossopharyngeal nerve, the canaliculus tympanicus, and the vomeronasal organ, which bear his name.

1783 ALEXANDER MONRO, Secundus of Edinburgh published
Observations on the Structure and Function of the Nervous System, discovered the communication between the lateral ventricles and the third ventricle of the brain (the foramen of Monro).

1784 Professor of anatomy from Italy, DOMENICO COTUGNO, observed and described cerebrospinal fluid (CSF) in fish and turtles, but was unable to detect it in humans.

1786 Crossing of fibers within the optic nerve (optic chiasma), a crescent-shaped grayish black nuclear material in the midbrain between the pedunculi and tegmentum (substantia nigra), and the long pudendal nerve, were described by SAMUEL THOMAS SÖMMERING, a German anatomist.

1787 JOHANNES EVANGELISTA PURKINJE born.
A physiologist from Czechoslovakia who studied visual phenomena and functioning of the brain (large nerve cells in the cerebral cortex) and heart (atypical myocardial fibers).

1789 Italian surgeon, ANTONIO SCARPA, gave one of the earliest and most comprehensive descriptions of the olfactory nerve.

1790 JOHANNES EHRENRITTER, a Viennese anatomist, described the ganglion of the glossopharyngeal nerve.

1790 The first report of central nervous system involvement in mumps was provided by ROBERT HAMILTON of Edinburgh in *An account of distemper in the common people of England, vulgarly called the mumps.*

1790 MARSHALL HALL born.
A British neurophysiologist who pioneered studies on artificial respiration (1855), and studied the nervous system and reflex activity of the medulla and spinal cord.

1791 JEAN CRUVEILHIER born.
A professor of pathology at Montpellier who gave the first description of disseminated or muscular sclerosis (1840), described a form of amyotrophic lateral sclerosis (Cruveilhier disease, 1853), and the regional lymph nodes.

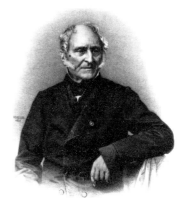

Jean Cruveilhier
(1791–1873)

1791 LUIGI GALVANI showed that electrical processes are involved in the function of muscles and nerves.

1793 ROBERT LEE born.
A Scottish physician at the Lying-in Hospital in London and lecturer at St George's Hospital, who accurately described the sympathetic ganglion of the cervix uteri (Lee ganglion) in 1842.

1793 MICHAEL UNDERWOOD, a London pediatrician, described a form of paralysis following a brief illness in children, probably the first scientific account of poliomyelitis.

1794 MARIE JEAN PIERRE FLOURENS born.
A French physiologist who was the first to perform extirpation of different parts of animal brains (1824), and later identified the respiratory center in the medulla oblongata (1837).

1795 MORITZ HEINRICH ROMBERG born.
A German professor of neurology who wrote the first formal treatise on nervous diseases, *Lehrbuch der Nervenkrankheiten* (1840), and described the pathognomonic sign in truncal sensory ataxia (Romberg sign).

1795 Facial paralysis was described by German physician, NIKOLAUS FRIEDRICH, SENIOR.

1797 JACOB SCHROEDER VAN DER KOLK born.
A physician from Utrecht who made microscopic studies of the medulla of the brain, and whose name is associated with the fibers of the reticular formation of the medulla.

1798 LOUIS FLORENTINE CALMIEL born.
A French physician who demonstrated the pathological lesions in the brain of patients with general syphilis.

1798 JOHN KEARSLEY MITCHELL born.
An American surgeon who wrote on mesmerism and neurology, and gave an original description of neurotic spinal arthropathies.

1799 ANTOINE LAURENT JESSIE BAYLE born.
A Paris physician who studied pathological lesions of the brain and described general paresis.

1799 CARL ADOLPH VON BASEDOW born.
A German physician who described Basedow syndrome, myeloneuropathy in thyrotoxicosis, and Basedow disease, thyrotoxicosis.

1799 SIR CHARLES LOCOCK born.
A British physician who suggested crowded teeth, onanism and menstruation as causes of epilepsy, for which he suggested treatment with potassium bromide.

1800 ALESSANDRO VOLTA investigated the effects of electricity on muscles.

1800 Gray matter was first interpreted as the active and functioning part of the brain by German physician, FRANZ JOSEPH GALL.

1801 JOHANNES PETER MÜLLER born.
A German physiologist who proposed the law of specific nerve energies (1840), and gave the first demonstration of the electrical nature of the heart (1855).

1801   RICHARD DUGARD GRAINGER born.
A British neurologist who demonstrated the role of gray
matter in the spinal cord in reflex activity (1837).

1801   CARL JOHANN CHRISTIAN GRAPENGIESSER of Berlin first used
galvanic current therapeutically.

1803   FRIEDRICH ARNOLD born.
An anatomist from Heidelberg who described the otic
ganglion of the 5th cranial nerve (Arnold ganglion).

1805   JOSEPH PANCOAST born.
A New Jersey anatomist and surgeon who performed a
section of the trigeminal nerve at the foramen ovale as
treatment for trigeminal neuralgia (1872), and published
A Treatise on Operative Surgery (1844).

1806   GUILLAUME BENJAMIN AMAND DUCHENNE born.
A physician from Paris and one of the earliest workers
on the electrophysiology of muscles. He described
Duchenne muscular dystrophy in early childhood,
different forms of lead palsy, and distinguished
rheumatic and lachrymal forms of facial paralysis from
brain or nerve lesions.

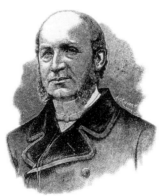

Guillaume Benjamin Amand Duchenne
(1806–1875)

1806 LUTHER V BELL born.
An American physician who described mania resulting from acute periencephalitis (Bell disease).

1807 ROBERT WILLIAM SMITH born.
A professor of surgery at Trinity College, Dublin who published a treatise on neurofibromatosis in 1849, *Treatise on the Pathology, Diagnosis, and Treatment of Neuroma*.

1807 FRANÇOIS LOUIS VALLEIX born.
A French physician who first described the tender points in a nerve causing neuralgia (Valleix points).

1808 Acute hydrocephalus was described by Scottish physician JOHN CHEYNE.

1808 ALEXANDER BAIN born.
A physician from Aberdeen, and a founder of modern systematic psychology who wrote *Senses and the Intellect* (1855) and *Emotions and the Will* (1859).

1809 JULES GABRIEL FRANÇOIS BAILLARGER born.
A French psychiatrist who described the internal and external lines of Baillarger in the cerebral cortex, and the bipolar illness with alternating states of depression and hypermania – manic depressive psychosis.

1809 Phrenic nerve palsy, a sign of thoracic aortic aneurysm, was described by Scottish surgeon and cardiologist, ALLAN BURNS, in *Observations of some of the Most Important and Frequent Diseases of the Heart*.

1810 DANIEL NOBLE born.
An English physician who published *The Human Mind in its Relationship with the Brain and Nervous System* (1858).

1810 American physician, NATHAN STRONG, gave one of the first and most important descriptions of cerebrospinal meningitis.

1810 LUDWIG TÜRCK born.
A Viennese neurologist who described the micropathology of the spinal cord in tabes dorsalis, and the direct pyramidal tracts in the Türck column (1856).

1811 The role of the ventral and dorsal roots of the spinal cord in reflex action was described by SIR CHARLES BELL, a Scottish anatomist and neurologist. He recognized that lesions of the 7th nerve could bring about facial palsy (Bell palsy, 1821), and wrote *Idea of a New Anatomy of the Brain*, in which he differentiated motor nerves and sensory nerves.

1811 ANDREA VERGA born.
An Italian neurologist from Milan who described a small tunnel in the petrous temporal bone between the corpus callosum and the body of Fornix (1856) which now bears his name.

1811 CARLO MATTEUCCI born.
An Italian physiologist who showed that current can be made to flow from the cut end of an isolated muscle to its uncut surface, if these points are connected by a galvanometer (1838).

1812   EDWARD SELLECK HARE born.
An English surgeon who gave an early description
of signs due to a cervical sympathetic lesion (Horner
syndrome, 1838).

1812   The respiratory center in the medulla oblongata was
discovered by a physician and physiologist from Brittany
in France, JULIEN JEAN CESAR LEGALLOIS.

1813   Delirium tremens, associated with alcoholism, was
described by THOMAS SUTTON of London.

1813   CLAUDE BERNARD born.
A celebrated French physiologist who established the
mechanism of vasomotor reflex responses (1851), and
introduced the concept of the internal environment of
the body (1865).

1813   Myotonic pupils and absent tendon reflexes, Adie
syndrome, was described by London ophthalmologist,
JAMES WARE.

1815   DANIEL CORNELIUS DANIELSSEN born.
A Norwegian physician who described Danielssen
disease, a form of anesthetic polyneuritis in leprosy.

1815   ROBERT REMAK born.
A German professor of neurology who noted that the gray
matter of the brain contained cellular tissue, described the
unmyelinated nerve fibers (Remak fibers, 1838), cardiac
ganglia (Remak ganglia, 1844), and classified the embryonic
germ layers.

1815 A minor form of epilepsy (petit mal) was described by JEAN ETIENNE DOMINIQUE ESQUIROL, a pioneer in mental disease from Toulouse in France. He studied states of dementia and was the first lecturer in psychiatry in Paris.

1816 AUGUSTUS VOLNEY WALLER born.
An English physiologist who demonstrated that the axis cylinder, if cut off from the nerve cell, will undergo degeneration while the stump will remain viable for a longer time (the law of Wallerian degeneration, 1850).

1816 LUDWIG MORITZ HIRSCHFELD born.
A Polish professor of anatomy who described the lingual branch of the facial nerve (Hirschfeld nerve) and the posterior renal sympathetic ganglion in 1866.

1816 EDWARD SIEVEKING born.
A British physician who produced a paper on epilepsy in *The Lancet*, including tested remedies.

1816 The point of emergence of the descending palatine nerve from the palato-maxillary canal (Méglin point) was described by French physician, J A MÉGLIN, an anatomist at Sultz.

1816 ALEXANDER ECKER born.
A German anatomist who provided an original description of several convolutions of the occipital lobe, and published works on the movement of the brain and spinal cord in 1843.

1817 CHARLES EDOUARD BROWN-SÉQUARD born.
A French-born American neurophysiologist who described hemiplegia associated with crossed anesthesia, Brown–Séquard syndrome (1850).

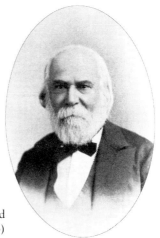

Charles Edouard Brown-Séquard
(1817–1894)

1817 The cavernous ganglion around the portion of the carotid artery within the cavernous sinus was described by Russian surgeon, AUGUST CARL BOCK.

1817 Parkinson disease, characterized by mask-like facies, tremor and slowness of movements, was described by London physician, JAMES PARKINSON.

1817 The first clear account of chronic subdural hematoma was given by M. HOUSSARD of Paris, although the condition had previously been observed at postmortem.

1817 JACOB AUGUSTUS CLARK born.
An eminent London neurologist who described the nucleus of the spinal cord (Clarke column), and the pigmented cells of the nucleus dorsalis (Clarke cells) in 1851.

1817 ETIENNE JULES BERGERON born.
A French physician who described hysterical chorea (Bergeron disease).

1817 KARL VOGT born.
A German neurophysiologist who defined the Vogt angle, found between the nasobasilar and alveolonasal lines.

1817 Nerve cells in the subthalamic nucleus (Pander cells) were described by German embryologist and anatomist, CHRISTIAN HEINRICH PANDER.

1817 WILHELM GRIESINGER born.
A neurologist from Germany who gave his name to the syndrome of pseudo-hypertrophic infantile muscular dystrophy.

1818 JEAN ANTOINE EUGÈNE BOUCHUT born.
A Paris physician who recognized the state of nervous exhaustion and asthenia (nervosisme) in 1860.

1818 LUDWIG TRAUBE born.
A German pathologist who worked on the pathology of fever and the effects of drugs on muscular activity, and described rhythmic variations of the vasoconstrictor center.

1818 EMIL DUBOIS-REYMOND born.
A professor of physiology in Berlin who demonstrated that the electrical state of the nerve altered when a current was passed through it, and described the injury potential of the muscle (1840).

1819 AUGUSTIN MARIE MORVAN born.
A French physician who described a form of syringomyelia with trophic changes in the extremities (Morvan disease).

1819 ERNST WILHELM VON BRÜCKE born.
One of Europe's leading physiologists who pioneered the functional study of phonetics, and described the luminosity of the eye by illuminating the fundus with artificial light.

1819 KARL WILHELM LUDWIG BRUCH born.
A German anatomist and professor at Giessen who described the lamina vitrea, a transparent membrane next to the retina separating it from the capillaries in the choroid (Bruch membrane, 1844).

1819 The posterior column of the spinal cord was described by CHARLES FREDERICK BURDACH, professor of medicine at Dorpat, Germany.

1820 A case of epilepsy associated with a remarkable slowness of the pulse, one of the first descriptions of heart block, was provided by English physician, WILLIAM BURNETT.

1821 Facial palsy arising from nuclear and infranuclear lesions of the facial nerve (Bell palsy) was described by Scottish neurologist, SIR CHARLES BELL, after original descriptions of the canal of the facial nerve by GABRIELE FALLOPPIO.

1821 HERMANN LUDWIG FERDINAND VON HELMHOLTZ born.
A German surgeon who developed a method of obtaining electromyograms (1851), carried out pioneering work on muscle energy (1850), and explained the mechanism of accommodation of the eye and perception of color.

1822   The first clear description of the functions of the facial nerve was given by English physician, HERBERT MAYO.

1822   Progressive paralysis of the insane (Bayle disease), pathological lesions of the brain, and general paresis, were described by French physician, ANTOINE LAURENT JESSE BAYLE.

1822   ADOLF KUSSMAUL born.
A German professor of surgery at Heidelberg who described cases of ascending neuropathy (1859), periarteritis nodosa (1866), progressive bulbar palsy (1873), and pulsus paradoxus (1873).

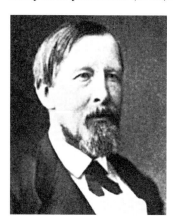

Adolf Kussmaul
(1822–1902)

1823   MORITZ SCHIFF born.
A German physiologist who defined the pathways for touch and pain sensations in the spinal cord.

1823   The idea that vision depends on the integrity of the cerebral cortex was established by French physiologist, PIERRE FLOURENS. He was the first to perform extirpation of different parts of animal brains and later identified the respiratory center in the medulla oblongata in 1824.

1824 PAUL BROCA born.
A French surgeon who located the motor area of speech in the 3rd frontal convolution of the brain (1861), and founded anthropometry with his inventions of 27 craniometric and cranioscopic instruments.

1824 Prostatoperitoneal aponeurosis (Tyrell fascia) was described by FREDERICK TYRELL, a surgeon at St Thomas' Hospital and nephew of SIR ASTLEY PASTON COOPER.

1824 Absence, a term describing a minor form of epilepsy, was coined by French physician, LOUIS FLORENTINE CALMIEL. He showed pathological lesions in the brain of patients with general paresis before the cause of syphilis was known.

1824 RICHARD LADISLAUS HESCHEL born.
A professor of anatomy at Olmutz who described the transverse gyri of the temporal lobes (1855).

1824 JOHANNES BERNHARD GUDDEN born.
A neuroanatomist from Munich who described the tract connecting the medial geniculate bodies and inferior corpora quadrigemina of the opposite side (1870), and pioneered physiological studies of the thalamus.

1825 NIKOLAUS FRIEDRICH born.
A German physician who wrote a significant treatise on progressive muscular atrophy, and described a hereditary spinocerebellar degenerative disease (Friedrich ataxia, 1863).

1825 JEAN-MARTIN CHARCOT born.
An eminent French neurologist who described tabetic arthropathies (Charcot joints), Charcot triad in multiple sclerosis, and osteoarthritis attributed to syphilis.

1825 The functions of cerebrospinal fluid (CSF) were elucidated by French physician, FRANÇOIS MAGENDIE, a founder of experimental physiology, who described the foramen of Magendie in 1828.

1826 EDMÉ FELIX ALFRED VULPIAN born.
A physician from Paris who demonstrated the presence of an active vital substance in the adrenal glands (1856), later named epinephrine, and described Vulpian atrophy in progressive muscular dystrophy.

1827 JEAN BAPTISTE CHAUVEAU born.
A French physiologist who pioneered the direct recording of cardiac impulses and the thermodynamics of muscular function.

1827 Trepanning as a treatment for bone necrosis and osteomyelitis were described by NATHAN SMITH, a surgeon from Connecticut.

1828 JULES BERNARD LUYS born.
A Paris neurologist who carried out research on hypnosis, hysteria and insanity, and described hemiballismus caused by lesions in the subthalamic body or the medial nucleus of the thalamus (nucleus of Luys).

1828 WILLIAM ALEXANDER HAMMOND born.
An American neurologist who wrote the first monograph on neurology in America, *Diseases of the Nervous System* (1871), described athetosis, carried out research on snake venom and arrow poisons, and was a founder of the American and New York Neurological Associations.

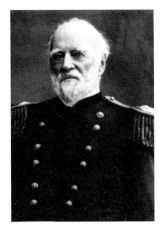

William Alexander Hammond
(1828–1900)

1828   JOHN SCOTT BURDON SANDERSON born.
A professor of medicine at Oxford who pioneered
electrophysiology, and devised an improved rheotome to study
the action currents of the heart.

1828   Probably the first description of a neuroma was given by
Scottish physician, WILLIAM WOOD.

1828   A description and illustration of the lesions in multiple
sclerosis was given by London pathologist, ROBERT HOOPER in
The Morbid Anatomy of the Human Brain.

1829   FRIEDRICH AUGUST KEKULE VON STRADONITZ born.
A German physician and organic chemist who, in his studies
of epilepsy, discovered the benzene ring structure that led to
the synthesis of phenobarbitone.

1829   JULES MARIE PARROT born.
A French physician who described the Parrot nodes on
the parietal and frontal bones of the skull of infants with
congenital syphilis (1879), and the Parrot sign, characterized
by dilatation of the pupils induced by pinching the skin of the
neck of patients with meningitis.

1829 FRIEDRICH GOLL born.
A neuroanatomist from Zurich who described fasciculus gracilis of the posterior column of the spinal cord (1868), and wrote *Minute Anatomy of the Spinal Cord of Man* in 1860.

1829 EDUARD FRIEDRICH WILHELM PFLÜGER born.
A German physiologist who carried out detailed studies of nerve stimulation, respiratory function, and discovered the Pflüger cords, a linear arrangement of sex cells during the development of the ovary (1863).

1830 SILAS WEIR MITCHELL born.
A Philadelphia neurologist who described a condition associated with painful feet, erythromelalgia (1872), demonstrated the knee jerk reflex (1886), and investigated the psychotic properties of mescaline (1896). He wrote *Injuries of the Nerves* in 1872.

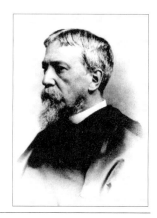

Silas Weir Mitchell
(1830–1914)

1830 WILLIAM BASIL NEFTEL born.
An American physician of Russian origin who described a hysterical disease in which the patient is unable to sit, stand or walk without pain, but can perform any movement lying down (Neftel disease).

1830 Salicin in willow bark as a mode of pain relief, was described by French physician, HENRI LEROUX.

1831 The first suggestion that herpes zoster was spread along a nerve was made by RICHARD BRIGHT of Guy's Hospital. He also first described changes in the brain in malaria.

1831 KARL VON VOIT born.
A German physiologist from Munich who described the cerebellar nucleus accessory to the corpus dentatum (Voit nucleus).

1831 CARL FRIEDRICH WILHELM FROMMANN born.
A professor of histology at Jena who demonstrated the striations in the axis cylinders of the nerve cell (Frommann striae, 1876), using silver nitrate stain.

1831 A classical description of delirium tremens was given by JOHN WARE, professor of medicine at Harvard University.

1831 ALARIK FRITHIOF HOLMGREN born.
A physiologist from Sweden who pioneered the application of electrophysiology to study visual systems, was the first to demonstrate retinal action currents, and developed the Holmgren test for color blindness.

1832 ERNST VICTOR VON LEYDEN born.
A German physician who worked on tabes and poliomyelitis, established sanatoria for treatment of tuberculosis, and described a form of muscular dystrophy (Leyden paralysis).

1832   WILHELM MAX WUNDT born.
An experimental psychologist from Germany who wrote
Beiträge zur Theorie der Sinneswahrnehmung, which highlighted
studies on voluntary reactions, reflex actions, and the theory
of sensory perception.

1832   ERNST AXLE HENRIK KEY born.
A Swedish professor of pathological anatomy who was one of
the first to describe the sensory nerve endings (Key bulb).

1832   SIR WILLIAM TURNER born.
A surgeon at Edinburgh University who described the
interparietal sulcus of the brain (Turner sulcus), and
wrote *The Convolutions of the Human Cerebrum Topographically
Considered* in 1864.

1832   Codeine, a base alkaloid of opium, was isolated by JEAN-
PIERRE ROBIQUET.

1833   The accessory ganglion of the great sympathetic system in
connection with the solar plexus (Lobstein ganglion), and
osteogenesis imperfecta (Lobstein syndrome) were described
by JOHANN GEORG LOBSTEIN, professor of pathology in
Strasburg.

1833   CARL FRIEDRICH OTTO WESTPHAL born.
A German neuropsychiatrist who described agoraphobia
(1871), demonstrated the absence of the knee jerk reflex in
tabes dorsalis (1875), and described the third cranial nerve
(Edinger–Westphal nucleus, 1887).

1833   Friedrich von Recklinghausen born.
A German pathologist who described a familial disease
marked by pedunculated soft tumors over the body
(neurofibromatosis, and multiple neuroma, or von
Recklinghausen disease, 1882).

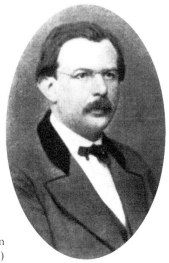

Friedrich von Recklinghausen
(1833–1910)

1833   Carl Jacob Christian Adolf Gerhardt born.
A professor from Germany who was a pioneer in pediatrics
and laryngology, and described bilateral adductor paralysis of
the larynx (1863).

1833   The segmented nature of the spinal cord and its interface
with the higher centers was demonstrated by British
neurophysiologist, Marshall Hall, who worked on
the nervous system and reflex activity of the medulla and
spinal cord.

1834   The first accurate description of tuberculous meningitis was
given by American physician, William Wood Gerhard.

1834 FRIEDRICH LEOPOLD GOLTZ born.
A German physiologist who pioneered work on vestibular disturbances and vertigo (1870), vagal reflex inhibition in relation to the heart, and showed the difference between cortical and subcortical functions.

1834 KARL EWALD KONSTANTIN HERING born.
A German physiologist who (with Joseph Breuer) described the Hering–Breuer neurogenic reflex controlling rate and depth of respiration via the vagal nerve (1868).

1834 VLADIMIR A BETZ born.
A Russian anatomist and histologist from Kiev who described the pyramidal cell in the 5th layer of the cerebral cortex (Betz cell, 1874).

1834 MARIE ERNST GELLÉ born.
A French surgeon and otologist who developed the Gellé test to demonstrate that deafness due to a bone conduction defect is not affected by pressure over the external auditory nerve.

1834 JOHN HUGHLINGS JACKSON born.
A British neurologist who established the use of the ophthalmoscope in brain disease, proposed that areas which caused specific isolated movements existed in the cortex (1864), and described a unilateral localized form of epilepsy.

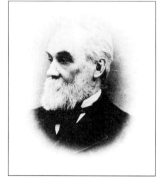

John Hughlings Jackson
(1834–1911)

1834 OTTO FRIEDRICH KARL DEITERS born.
A German physician and histologist who made several
contributions in neuro-auditory anatomy and the
structure of the internal ear, and also described the
lateral vestibular nucleus (Deiters nucleus, 1863).

1834 SOLOMON STRICKER born.
A German physician who, in studies on the treatment of
pain relief, discovered that sodium salicylic acid arrests
rheumatic fever.

1834 H M D DE BLAINVILLE of Paris demonstrated massive
intravascular clotting in experimental animals, following an
intravenous injection of brain tissue.

1835 THOMAS GEORGE MORTON born.
An American surgeon from Philadelphia who gave a complete
description of metatarsalgia with neuralgia of the lateral
plantar nerve (Morton disease, 1876).

1835 LOUIS ANTHOINE RANVIER born.
A French physician who made a special study of the peripheral
nerves, and described the regular interruptions of the myelin
sheath (nodes of Ranvier, 1878).

1835 SIR WILLIAM HENRY BROADBENT born.
An eminent neurologist from England who proposed the
Broadbent hypothesis for the recovery of motor power of the
muscles in paralysis, and described apoplexy due to cerebral
hemorrhage in the ventricles.

1835   VALENTIN JACQUES JOSEPH MAGNAN born.
A French psychiatrist and one of the leaders in the
school of organic psychiatry, who described the crawling
sensation under the skin in cocaine addiction (Magnan
sign).

1835   FRANTISEK CHVOSTEK born.
An Austrian surgeon from Moravia who investigated
pathology and treatment of neurological illnesses,
including the use of electrotherapy, and described the
Chvostek sign of facial spasm in tetany (1876).

1835   MORITZ BENEDIKT born.
A Hungarian-born Austrian physician who used electricity for
the treatment of diseases, and gave his name to Benedikt
syndrome of paralysis of the oculomotor nerve with tremors
and ataxia on the contralateral side (1889).

1835   RUDOLF ARNDT born.
A German psychiatrist who proposed the idea that weak
stimuli cause strong physiological responses and strong
stimuli diminish physiological activity (Arndt–Schultz
law).

1836   SIR THOMAS CLIFFORD ALLBUTT born.
An English physician who gave an early description of
joint symptoms in locomotor ataxia (1858), and studied
the effects of strain in producing heart diseases and
aneurysms.

1836   Thirty-nine cases of lead encephalopathy were
published by AUGUSTIN GRISOLLE of Paris who divided
them into convulsive, comatosed, and delirious states.

1836 HEINRICH WILHELM GOTTFRIED WALDEYER(-HARTZ) born.
A German histologist who gave a histological
classification of cancers showing that carcinomas come
from epithelial cells and sarcomas from mesodermal
tissue. He suggested the terms 'chromosome', 'neuron'
and 'motor neuron' in 1891.

1836 ALBERT VON BEZOLD born.
A German physiologist who discovered the accelerator
nerve fibers of the heart and their origin in the spinal
cord (1862), and described the Bezold ganglia in the
interauricular system (1863).

1836 Myelinated nerve fibers were differentiated from the
unsheathed fibers by CHRISTIAN GOTTFRIED EHRENBERG of
Germany.

1837 The English physician, THOMAS ADDISON, was the first to use
static electricity in the treatment of nervous diseases.

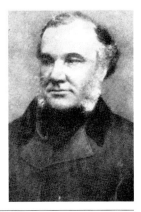

Thomas Addison
(1793–1860)

1837 The role of gray matter in the spinal cord in reflex
activity was shown by RICHARD DUGARD GRAINGER, a
British neurologist.

1837 HENRY CHARLTON BASTIAN born.
One of the founders of British neurology who described the abolition of tendon reflexes in the lower extremities, associated with lesions above the lumbar segment of the spinal cord (Bastian law), and wrote *Aphasia and Other Speech Defects* in 1898, and *The Brain as an Organ of the Mind*.

1837 British neurophysiologist, MARSHALL HALL, produced treatises on the medulla oblongata, medulla spinalis, and on the oxitomotor system of nerves.

1837 BERTHOLD STILLER born.
A Hungarian physician who described general asthenia (Stiller disease) in 1907.

1837 WILLIAM KEEN born.
Regarded as America's first brain surgeon, he successfully removed a meningioma (1888), tapped the ventricles (1889), and published a *System of Surgery* in eight volumes from 1906 to 1921.

1837 French physiologist, PIERRE FLOURENS, showed that by identifying and inducing a lesion in the bilateral 'vital nodes' of the respiratory centers of the medulla oblongata, asphyxia was produced.

1837 WILHELM KÜHNE born.
A German biochemist and physiologist who discovered the visual purple in the retina (rhodopsin), and described the neuromuscular spindle (Kühne spindle, 1862).

1838 THEODOR FRITSCH born.
A military surgeon during the Prussian–Danish war who did experiments on stimulation of the brain, proving the existence of motor control areas in the cerebral cortex (published in 1870).

1838 JULIUS EDUARD HITZIG born.
A German neurologist who worked with THEODOR FRITSCH and experimented on the stimulation of the brain using dogs, and showed that stimulation of the motor cortex produced movements on the opposite side of the body.

1838 CHARLES HILTON FAGGE born.
A physician at Guy's Hospital, London who described sporadic cretinism, ankylosing spondylitis and gave an exhaustive account of presystolic murmurs.

1838 Inhibition of the heart by stimulating the vagus nerve was demonstrated by ALFRED WILHELM VOLKMANN, a surgeon from Germany, who also experimentally induced bronchospasm by stimulation six years later.

1838 Curare was first used in medical practice to relax the muscles in rabies.

1839 JULIUS BERNSTEIN born.
A German professor of physiology who invented a differential rheotome to record voluntary muscle contraction, and proposed the cell membrane theory to explain the electrical properties of muscles (1912).

1839 WILLIAM RUTHERFORD born.
A Scottish professor of physiology who pioneered the study of hearing, and proposed that the tympanic membrane receiving the sound vibrated like a microphone and imparted electrical impulses to the brain.

1839 The thin membranous outer covering of the myelin sheath of the nerve fiber (sheath of Schwann) was described and named by THEODOR SCHWANN, professor of anatomy and physiology at Liege, Belgium.

1839 CHARLES H HUGHES born.
An American neurologist who founded the *Journal of Neurology and Psychiatry*, and gave his name to the Hughes reflex, the downward movement of the penis when the glans or prepuce are pulled upwards.

1839 JULIUS FRIEDRICH COHNHEIM born.
A German pathologist who pioneered histology and pathology in his dissertation on inflammation of the serous membranes, and introduced silver staining of nerve endings in muscles.

1839 KARL HUGO KRONECKER born.
A German physiologist who described the swallowing reflex involved in the act of deglutition, and a cardio-inhibitory center (Kronecker center).

1839 The Valentin ganglion, situated on the superior dental nerve, was described by a professor of physiology at Bern, Switzerland, GABRIEL GUSTAV VALENTIN.

1840   JOHN DIXON MANN born.
A Manchester physician who described a change in electrical resistance of the skin thought to be associated with certain neuroses.

1840   LUDWIG MAUTHNER born.
A professor of ophthalmology in Vienna who described the membrane surrounding the axis of the nerve within the sheath of Schwann (Mauthner membrane, 1860).

1840   Sensory nerve end organs (Pacini corpuscles) were described by Italian professor of anatomy at Pisa, FILIPPO PACINI.

1840   WILHELM HEINRICH ERB born.
A German neurologist who described brachial palsy (1874), syphilitic spinal paralysis (1875), discovered the absence of knee jerk in spinal syphilis, and developed electrotherapy as treatment for nervous diseases (1882).

1840   HENRY PICKERING BOWDITCH born.
A Boston physiologist who carried out important studies on the physiology of the heart muscles and nerves, including the increase in heart rate having a positive inotropic effect (Bowditch effect), and experimented on nerve block.

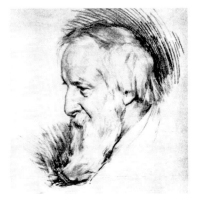

Henry Pickering Bowditch
(1840–1911)

1840 SIR DYCE DUCKWORTH born.
A London physician who described the occurrence of
respiratory before cardiac arrest in certain cases of brain
infection (Duckworth phenomenon).

1840 CARLO GIACOMO born.
A professor of anatomy and neurologist in Turin who
gave original descriptions of several neuroanatomical
structures.

1840 French psychiatrist, JULES GABRIEL FRANÇOIS BAILLARGER,
noted the line of Gennari in the cerebral cortex
that consists of two bands separated by a thin dark
line (Baillarger lines). He described a bipolar illness with
alternating states of depression and hypermania – manic
depressive psychosis.

1840 One of the first descriptions of infantile paralysis was given by
German orthopedic surgeon, JACOB VON HEINE.

1840 VLADIMIR MICHAILOVICH KERNIG born.
A Russian neurologist who described how flexion of the thigh
at the hip and extension of the leg causes pain and spasm in
the hamstrings in cases of meningitis or encephalitis (Kernig
sign, 1909).

1840 The first modern treatise on neurology, *Lehrbuch der
Nerven-Krankheiten*, was written by MORITZ HEINRICH
ROMBERG of Berlin, who also described the
pathognomonic sign in truncal sensory ataxia (Romberg sign).

1840   DÉSIRÉ MAGLOIRE BOURNEVILLE born.
A French neurologist who described adenoma sebaceum associated with mental deficiency and epilepsy (1880), made observations on cretinism, mongolism and myxedema, and established the first school for mentally defective children.

1840   The paralyzing effect of curare on the myoneural junction in frogs was demonstrated by French physiologist, CLAUDE BERNARD.

1840   LUIGI LUCIANI born.
An Italian physician and professor of physiology at Siena, Florence and Rome who described hypotonia, ataxia and weakness seen in cerebellar disease (Luciani triad).

1841   The ciliospinal and genitospinal centers of the spinal cord were described by JULIUS LUDWIG BUDGE, a professor of physiology from Bonn, Germany.

1841   GUSTAV HUGENIN born.
A professor of psychiatry at Zurich who described a system of levels for motor and sensory neurons (1879).

1841   CARL HERMAN WILHELM NOTHNAGEL born.
A German physician who described unilateral oculomotor paralysis associated with ipsilateral ataxia, due to lesions of the superior cerebral peduncle of the brain (Northnagel paralysis).

1841   LOUIS HUBERT FARABEUF born.
A professor of anatomy at the Faculty of Medicine in
Paris who described the triangle in the upper part of the
neck, bounded by the internal jugular vein, the facial
vein, and the hypoglossal nerve, and later named after
him.

1841   EMIL THEODOR KOCHER born.
A professor of surgery from Switzerland and Nobel laureate
(1909) who pioneered methods of brain and spinal cord
surgery, and devised an operation for the reduction of
subluxation of the shoulder joint.

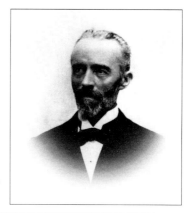

Emil Theodor Kocher
(1841–1917)

1842   The autonomic nervous system was investigated by
German anatomist at Dorpat, FRIEDRICH HEINRICH
WILHELM BIDDER, who showed that it contained small
medullated fibers from the spinal and sympathetic
ganglia.

1842   RICHARD CATON born.
An English physician who detected and identified electric
activity in the brain of living animals.

1842 CHARLES ABADIE born.
A French ophthalmologist at L'Hôtel Dieu who introduced alcohol injection of the Gasserian ganglion to treat trigeminal neuralgia, and described spasm of the levator palprebrae muscle of the eye in exophthalamic goiter (1877).

1842 HEINRICH IRANAEUS QUINCKE born.
A German professor of medicine at Bern in Switzerland, who gave an account of angioneurotic edema (1882), and performed therapeutic lumbar puncture (1891).

1842 MAGNUS GUSTAV RETZIUS born.
A Swedish neuroanatomist who described the brown lines in the enamel of teeth, known as striae of Retzius (1890), and whose name is associated with several structures of the brain.

1842 FRANÇOIS HENRI HALLIPEAU born.
A French dermatologist who described a variant of Neumann pemphigus vegetans (Hallipeau disease, 1889), and wrote theses on diseases of the spinal cord, diffuse myelitis and bulbar palsy.

1842 GEORGE TRUMBELL LADD born.
An American psychologist and professor of philosophy at Yale who studied the relationship between the nervous system and mental phenomena, and published *Elements of Physiological Psychology* (1887).

1842 The earliest description of hereditary chorea was given by American physician, ROBLEY DUNGLISON.

1843 CAMILLO GOLGI born.
An Italian neurologist and Nobel Prize winner (1906) who described motor units, sensory cells, the tactile Golgi end-organs, named 'axons' and 'dendrites', and developed several staining techniques for nerve tissue.

1843 A study of the nervous control of the circulatory system was carried out by French physiologist, CLAUDE BERNARD.

1843 SIR DAVID FERRIER born.
A Scottish neurologist who was a pioneer in the study of localization of cerebral function, wrote *Functions of the Brain* (1876) and *Localization of the Cerebral Disease* (1878), and was founding editor of the journal *Brain*.

1844 German neurologist, ROBERT REMAK, discovered the cardiac ganglia (Remak ganglia), noted that gray matter of the brain contained cellular tissue, and described unmyelinated nerve fibers (Remak fibers).

1844 FRANÇOIS ALEXIS ALBERT GOMBAULT born.
A neuropathologist from Paris who gave original descriptions of several tracts in the spinal cord in his *Etude sur la Sclerose Laterale Amylotrophique* (1870).

1844 GUSTAV ALBERT SCHWALBE born.
A German neuroanatomist who described the vestibular nucleus and several other structures of the brain which are named after him.

1845 German physiologists (and brothers), FRIEDRICH WEBER and ERNST HEINRICH WEBER, demonstrated the inhibitory effects of the vagus nerve on the heart.

1845 Prostatoperitoneal aponeurosis was described by CHARLES PIERRE DENONVILLIERS, professor of surgery and anatomy from Paris.

1845 CHARLES KARSNER MILLS born.
An early professor of neurology at the University of Pennsylvania who described unilateral progressive ascending paralysis (Mills disease, 1900).

1845 ANTON WEICHELSBAUM born.
An Austrian pathologist who isolated meningococcus or *Diplococcus intercellularis meningitides* from the cerebrospinal fluid of patients with meningitis in 1887.

1845 KARL WEIGERT born.
A German pathologist who devised some of the earliest and best staining methods for bacteria and tissues (myelin sheath in 1884 and elastic fibers in 1898), and described the pathological anatomy in Bright disease (1879).

1845 EMIL HEINRICH DUBOIS-REYMOND, a German professor of physiology from Berlin, demonstrated the existence of resting current in nerves.

1845 FRIEDRICH SIGMUND MERKEL born.
A German anatomist who described sensory tactile nerve endings in the skin (Merkel corpuscles, 1880), and the meniscus tactus.

1846   RICHARD CLEMENT LUCAS born.
A surgeon at Guy's Hospital who was the first to describe the
groove made by the chorda tympani nerve on the spine of the
sphenoid (Lucas groove, 1894).

1846   HANS CURSCHMANN born.
A German physician who described the spiral threads of
mucus expectorated by an asthmatic (Curschmann spirals)
and a rare hereditary syndrome with myotonia of lingual and
thenar muscles (Curschmann–Batten– Steinert syndrome,
1912).

1846   Classic research on cerebral circulation was published by
London physician, GEORGE BURROWES in *On the Disorders of
the Cerebral Circulation and the Connections between the
Affections of the Brain and Diseases of the Heart*.

1846   FELIX JACOB MARCHAND born.
A German pathologist who used a crude differential rheotome
connected to a galvanometer to measure the electrical
variation of a frog's heart (1872), and introduced the term
'atherosclerosis' in 1904.

1846   JAMES JACKSON PUTNAM born.
A Harvard neurologist who studied
circumscribed analgesia, neuritis from lead
poisoning, polio, myxedema and spinal
cord tumors. He was a founder of the
American Neurological Association.

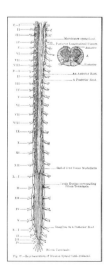

Nerves in the
spinal cord

1847   WILLIAM BEVAN-LEWIS born.
A professor of mental diseases at Leeds who described the large cells of the motor cortex (Bevan-Lewis cells, 1879).

1847   PAUL FREDERICK EMMANUEL VOGT born.
A German surgeon who defined the Vogt point in the skull where trephination can be performed for traumatic meningeal hemorrhage.

1847   WILLIAM ROSE born.
An English surgeon who performed excision of the Gasserian ganglion as treatment for trigeminal neuralgia.

1847   PAUL EMIL FLECHSIG born.
A German neurologist who mapped the brain, was the first to describe auditory radiation, and the dorsal spinocerebellar tract (Flechsig tract).

1847   ISAAC OTT born.
An American physician who carried out extensive work on nervous regulation of body temperature for over 30 years, leading to the discovery of the thermoregulatory center in the hypothalamus.

1847   WALTER HOLBROOK GASKELL born.
An English physiologist who introduced the term 'block' in cardiology, described the accelerator nerves of the heart (1881), and laid the foundation for understanding the autonomic nervous system.

1847   VIRGIL PENDLETON GIBNEY born.
A New York surgeon who described painful fibrositis of the spinal muscles (Gibney perispondylitis).

1847   Hans Christian Saxtroph Helvig born.
A psychiatrist and director of the Institute for the Insane in Odense who described the tractus-olivospinalis of the nervous system (1887).

1847   The symptoms and signs of tabes dorsalis (locomotor ataxia) were given by British physician, Robert Bentley Todd of King's College, London.

1848   Leonardo Bianchi born.
An Italian neuropsychiatrist who described Bianchi syndrome, sensory aphasia accompanied by alexia and apraxia, and seen in lesions of the left parietal lobe.

1848   Jean Albert Pitres born.
A French physician who defined several specific areas in the prefrontal cortex, the Pitres areas.

1848   Vladimir Karlovitch Roth born.
A Russian neurologist who described septic retinitis (Roth disease).

1848   Auguste Forel born.
A professor of psychiatry at Zurich who pioneered the study of subthalamic areas of the central nervous system, described decussation between the red nuclei of the brain (Forel decussation), and wrote *The Sexual Problem* in 1905.

1848   Carl Furstner born.
A German psychiatrist who described pseudospastic paralysis with tremors (Furstner disease).

1848   ALEXANDER HUGHES BENNET born.
An English neurologist who performed the diagnosis and
operative removal of a brain tumor in 1884.

1848   KARL WERNICKE born.
A German neurologist who described Wernicke
encephalopathy, ophthalmoplegia, nystagmus, ataxia with
tremors from thiamin deficiency, and aphasia, and the
Wernicke area, a sensory speech center.

1848   SIR WILLIAM MACEWEN born.
A professor of surgery from Scotland who was one of the first
to successfully operate on brain tumors, abscesses and trauma,
and removed a tumor involving the meninges of the brain
(1879).

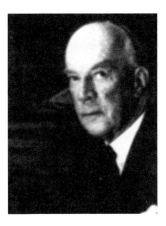

Sir William Macewen
(1848–1924)

1849   JOSEPH GRASSET born.
A French neurologist who described the drawing of the head
to the side in cases of unilateral cerebral lesions, producing
flaccid hemiplegia (Grasset law).

1849 French neurologist, GUILLAUME DUCHENNE, described progressive spinal muscular atrophy, Aran–Duchenne disease, Duchenne muscular dystrophy in early childhood, differing forms of lead palsy, and distinguished rheumatic and lachrymal forms of facial paralysis from brain or nerve lesions.

1849 HENRY DURET born.
A French neurosurgeon who described the arteries supplying the nuclei of the cranial nerves and the subarachnoid canals.

1849 Multiple neurofibromatosis was originally described by ROBERT WILLIAM SMITH from Dublin in his *Treatise on Pathology, Diagnosis and Treatment of Neuroma*. It was later named von Recklinghausen disease, although Smith's description was 33 years earlier.

1849 HERMANN EICHORST born.
A physician from Zurich who described a type of progressive muscular atrophy affecting the femoral and tibial muscles.

1849 CHARLES ÉMILE FRANÇOIS FRANCK born.
A French physiologist and neurologist who carried out studies on the excitability of the cerebral cortex, and localization of its activity.

1849 German neurologist, ROBERT REMAK, discovered the Remak reflex in spinal cord lesions, Remak paralysis in lead poisoning, and carried out work on the peripheral nerves and neuropathies.

1849 OTTO KAHLER born.
A German physician who described the course of the posterior nerve roots that enter the posterior columns, so that fibers at higher levels medially displace those from lower levels, and also gave a description of multiple myeloma (Kahler–Pick law).

1849 AUGUST FRORIEP born.
A physiologist from Tübingen who described a dorsal root ganglion (Froriep ganglion) found inconsistently at a position posterior to the hypoglossal nerve.

1849 IVAN PETROVITCH PAVLOV born.
An experimental physiologist from central Russia who discovered the secretory nerves of the pancreas (1888), worked on the circulatory system, digestive glands and conditioned reflexes, and was awarded the Nobel Prize in 1904.

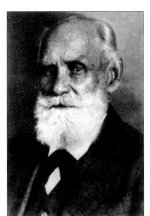

Ivan Petrovitch Pavlov
(1849–1936)

1849 FRANZ CHRISTIAN BOLL born.
A Swiss anatomist who discovered the basal cells of the lachrymal glands (1869), and the photosensitive pigment in the retina (rhodopsin, 1877).

1849 SIR WILLIAM OSLER born.
Regius professor of medicine at Oxford, originally from
Canada, who described effective treatment of Addison disease
(1896), hereditary angioneurotic edema (1888), familial
hemorrhagic telengiectasis (1907), wrote *Principles and Practice
of Medicine,* and reformed American medical education.

1850 ADAM ADAMKIEWICZ born.
A Polish pathologist who described a branch of the abdominal
aorta that supplies the spinal cord below the level of L1
(artery of Adamkiewicz, 1882).

1850 Amyotrophic lateral sclerosis was described by FRANÇOIS
AMILCAR ARAN as progressive muscular atrophy.

1850 GEORGE HUNTINGTON born.
An American neurologist who was the first to recognize adult
hereditary (Huntington) chorea, and to detail its symptoms in
1872.

1850 SIR EDWARD SHARPEY-SCHÄFER born.
A pioneer in endocrinology who demonstrated the effects of
suprarenal gland extract (epinephrine) and showed that it
produced artery contraction and accelerated heart rate, thus
increasing blood pressure.

1850 An instrument for determining the velocity of a nerve
current (myographion) was invented by German professor
of physiology, HERMANN VON HELMHOLTZ. He did pioneering
work on muscle energy and invented an ophthalmoscope.
In 1852 he showed that the maximum velocity of nerve
conduction in experimental animals was 30 meters
per second.

1850   IVAN MICHAILOVITCH SETCHENOV born.
Considered the father of Russian physiology and neurology, he described the reflex inhibitory center in the medulla oblongata (Setchenov center), and several other structures of the nervous system.

1850   Retinal changes in hypertension were observed by Viennese neurologist, LUDWIG TÜRCK.

1850   Surgical treatment of a cerebral abscess by opening the lateral ventricles was performed by WILLIAM DETMOLD of America.

1850   Multiple myeloma or myelomatosis was described by English physician, WILLIAM MACINTYRE.

1850   The deterioration of mental processes from adolescence (presenile dementia) was first observed by French psychiatrist, AUGUSTIN BENTOIT MOREL, who named it demence precoce.

1850   GERARD MARCHANT born.
A French surgeon who described the points of easily detachable connections of the dura mater to the basal, sphenoidal, and occipital bones of the skull (Marchant zone, 1881).

1851   Nerves of the salivary glands were described by German physiologist, KARL WILHELM LUDWIG. He invented a Kymograph to measure circulation and respiration (1846), a blood pump (1859), and a steam gauge (1867).

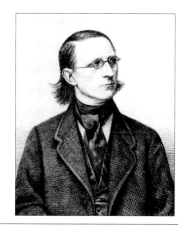

Karl Wilhelm Ludwig
(1816–1895)

1852   SAMUEL VULFOVICH GOLDFLAM born.
A neurologist working in Warsaw who described myasthenia gravis in 1893.

1852   EDWARD CHARLES SPITZKA born.
A New York neurologist who described the fibers of the posterior longitudinal bundle connecting the 3rd and 6th nerve cranial nuclei (bundle of Spitzka, 1876), and was editor of the *American Journal of Neurology*.

1852   THEODOR KAES born.
A neurologist from Germany who described a new layer in the cerebral cortex (Kaes–Bekhterev layer, 1907), with Russian neurologist VLADIMIR MIKHAILOVITCH BEKHTEREV.

1852   MAX SCHÄFFER born.
A German physician who described the extension of the great toe on pinching the achilles tendon (Schäffer reflex).

1852   EDOUARD BRISSAUD born.
A French neurologist who described infantile myxedema (1907), and a condition of uncontrolled tic spasms in children (1896).

1852 GUILLAUME VIGNAL born.
A French histologist who described the embryonic connective tissue on the axis cylinders of fetal nerve fibers (Vignal cells, 1889).

1852 SANTIAGO RAMON Y CAJAL born.
A Spanish physician, Nobel laureate (1906), and a professor of anatomy in Valencia and Barcelona, who studied the microstructure of the nervous system (including nerve degeneration and regeneration), and developed many histological stains.

1852 Tactile sensory nerve endings (Meissner corpuscles) were described by GEORG MEISSNER and RUDOLF WAGNER, professors of physiology at Göttingen, Germany.

1852 CHARLES LOOMES DANA born.
A New York neurologist who designed an operation for resection of the posterior roots of the spinal nerves as treatment for intractable pain, athetosis, or spastic paralysis (Dana operation, 1891).

1852 JOHN NEWPORT LANGLEY born.
A neurophysiologist from Newbury, England who coined the terms 'preganglionic', 'postganglionic' and 'autonomic' during work on the nervous system, and wrote *The Autonomic Nervous System* in 1921.

1852 The ganglionic cells (Bidder ganglia) at the junction of the auricles and ventricles were discovered by German anatomist, FRIEDRICH HEINRICH BIDDER.

1852   Alexander Stanislavovic Dogiel born.
A Russian neurologist who described nerve endings of the
bulb type (1903), and created a classification of spinal and
other ganglia.

1853   Sir Frederick Treves born.
An English surgeon who wrote *The Elephant Man and
other Reminiscences*, the true story of Joseph Merrick, a grossly
deformed man suffering from neurofibromatosis.

1853   Robert Adolf Tigerstedt born.
A physiologist from Finland who discovered pressor substance
(renin) in the kidneys and discharged into the circulation of
the renal glands, and carried out studies on nerve response to
mechanical stimulation.

1853   Sir James Mackenzie born.
One of the greatest British cardiologists who noted the loss of
effective atrial contraction (atrial paralysis), described the
functional pathology of cardiac tissue, and published *Diseases
of the Heart*.

1853   Gilbert Ballet born.
A Paris physician who described Ballet disease, paralysis
of the extraocular muscles in cases of thyrotoxic
exophthalmos.

1853   Wilhelm Uhthoff born.
A German physician and ophthalmologist who described the
occurrence of nystagmus in multiple sclerosis (Uhthoff sign).

1854 SERGEI SERGEIVICH KORSAKOFF born.
A Russian neurologist and neuropsychiatrist who described alcoholic polyneuritis (1887) and Korsakoff psychosis.

1854 Neuroglia, the supporting structures of the nerve tissue, were described by German pathological anatomist, RUDOLPH VIRCHOW, and in 1856 he published *Die Cellularpathologie*.

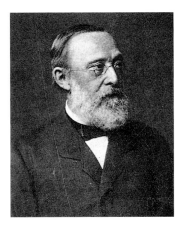

Rudolph Virchow
(1821–1902)

1854 The center of the brain, acting as the 'master switchboard' for controlling and regulating the circulatory system was located by CARL FRIEDRICH LUDWIG.

1854 ARNALDO ANGELUCCI born.
An Italian ophthalmologist who described vernal conjunctivitis, hyperexcitability, tachycardia and vasomotor liability (Angelucci syndrome), and maintained a life-long interest in trachoma.

1854 PHILLIPE CHARLES ERNEST GAUCHER born.
A French physician who described a disorder of
cerebroside metabolism with large pale cells in the
spleen, as 'epithelioma primitif de la rate' (Gaucher
disease, 1882).

1855 LUDWIG EDINGER born.
A German anatomist and a founder of comparative
neuroanatomy, who described the nucleus of the third
cranial nerve, the Edinger–Westphal nucleus (1885).

1855 EMIL BERGER born.
An Austrian ophthalmologist who described irregular
pupils (Berger sign) in cases of early neurosyphilis.

1855 The symptomology of tabes dorsalis (locomotor ataxia) was
described by SIR JOHN RUSSELL REYNOLDS, professor of
medicine in London, in his *Diagnosis of the Diseases of
the Spinal Cord and Nerves*.

1855 The Luschka foramen at the lateral recesses of the 4th
ventricle of the brain, was described by HUBERT VON LUSCHKA
(1855), professor of anatomy at Tübingen.

1855 British neurophysiologist, MARSHALL HALL, devised a method
of artificial respiration.

1855 The adrenals were removed by EDOUARD BROWN-SÉQUARD, a
French physician and neurologist, who found them essential
to life, and with a detoxicating effect.

1855 Brachial palsy (Erb palsy) was described by the English
obstetrician, WILLIAM SMELLIE and French neurologist,
GUILLAUME DUCHENNE.

1855 JAMES LEONARD CORNING born.
A New York physician who produced a block of nerve roots between the dura mater and the vertebral canal as a form of regional anesthesia (extradural block, 1885).

1855 The Rinnie test, using a tuning fork to differentiate between sensorimotor deafness and conduction deafness, was devised by German otologist, HEINRICH ADOLF RINNIE.

1855 GEORGE EDOUARD ALBERT GILLES DE LA TOURETTE born.
A French neurologist who described a syndrome of violent muscle jerks of the face, shoulders, and extremities (Tourette syndrome, 1885), and worked on hysteria and hypnotism.

1856 Interference of the vascular blood supply to the pons, causing abducens and facial nerve paralysis with contralateral hemiplegia (Millard–Gubler syndrome) was described by French physicians, ADOLPHE GUBLER and AUGUSTE MILLARD.

1856 The ganglion around the cochlear nerve within the internal auditory meatus was described by ARTHUR BÖTTCHER.

1856 Paraplegia was studied at postmortem by SIR WILLIAM GULL of Guy's Hospital, London. He described the cretinoid state in the adult (Gull disease) or myxedema (in a woman).

1856 French physiologist, CLAUDE BERNARD, demonstrated the neuromuscular blocking effect of curare, and in 1858 he discovered the vasodilator fibers in the chorda tympani.

1856 Epileptic hemiplegia affecting the epileptic side (Todd paralysis) was described by ROBERT BENTLEY TODD, an English physician and professor of physiology at King's College.

1856 HOWARD HENRY TOOTH born.
An English physician who described the peroneal form of progressive muscular dystrophy (Charcot–Marie–Tooth–Hoffmann syndrome, 1886).

1857 SIR VICTOR ALEXANDER HADEN HORSLEY born.
The founder of neurosurgery in Britain who proved that myxedema and cretinism are due to thyroid deficiency (1886), performed the first successful removal of a spinal tumor (1887), and produced a stereotactic apparatus for accurate location of electrodes in the brain (1908).

1857 SIR CHARLES SCOTT SHERRINGTON born.
An English physiologist and neurologist who demonstrated decerebrate rigidity by transection of the spinal cord through the upper part of the midbrain (1897), established the knee jerk reflex as an inherited phenomenon (1893), and first used the term 'motor unit' (1925).

1857 HENDRICK ZWAARDEMAKER born.
A German physiologist who made careful and detailed studies on functional aspects of the sense of smell.

1857 JULIUS WAGNER-JAUREGG born.
An Austrian neurologist and Nobel laureate (1927) who investigated the relationship between cretinism and goiter, and treated late stage paralysis in syphilis by inducing malarial fever.

1857   VLADIMIR M BEKHTEREV born.
A Russian neurologist who studied brain morphology, discovered the superior vestibular nucleus, described numbness of the spine, and a new form of spondylitis (1897).

1857   FEDOR VICTOR KRAUSE born.
A Berlin surgeon who described the Krause operation for trigeminal neuralgia, involving extra-dural excision of the Gasserian ganglion.

1857   British physician SIR CHARLES LOCOCK first used bromide in treatment of epilepsy.

1858   BERNARD PARNEY SACHS born.
An American neurologist who worked on mental and nervous diseases, wrote on amaurotic familial idiocy, and published *Nervous Diseases of Children*. He and WARREN TAY described amaurotic idiocy (a gangliosidosis) – Tay–Sachs disease.

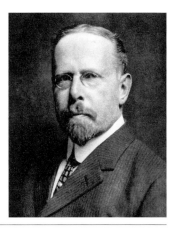

Bernard Parney Sachs
(1858–1944)

1858   French neurologist, ACHILLE LOUIS FOVILLE, gave his name to Foville syndrome, abducens and facial nerve paralysis with contralateral hemiplegia due to a pontine lesion.

1858   LUDWIG BRUNS born.
A German neurologist from Hannover who described
vertigo as a result of sudden movements of the head, caused
by cystisclerosis of the 4th ventricle in the brain (Bruns
syndrome).

1858   Tabes dorsalis was described as 'locomotor ataxy' by
GUILLAUME DUCHENNE, an eminent neurologist from Paris.

1858   JOHANNES KARL EUGEN ALFRED GOLDSCHEIDER born.
A German neurologist who gave a complete description of
epidermolysis bullosa (Goldscheider disease, 1882).

1858   HAROLD GIFFORD born.
An American ophthalmologist who described
constriction of the pupils occurring when the orbicularis
occuli muscle is contracted with open eyelids
(Gifford reflex).

1858   Contraction of heart muscle accompanied by electrical
activity originating in the heart muscle (electrocardiography)
was demonstrated by Swiss physiologist KÖLLIKER and
German anatomist, MÜLLER.

1858   French physiologist, CLAUDE BERNARD, discovered the
vasodilator fibers in the chorda tympani, and demonstrated an
increase in blood flow to the area on stimulation.

1858   GABRIEL ANTON born.
An Austrian neurologist who linked brain pathology with
psychology in pioneering work on lack of self-perception of
deficits in patients with cortical blindness and deafness,
Anton syndrome (1899).

1858   MAX FRIEDMANN born.
A German physician who described a form of relapsing
infantile spinal paralysis (Friedmann disease).

1859   The National Hospital for the Relief of Paralysis,
Epilepsy and Allied Disorders, the first neurological
center in the world, was started in London by
LOUISA CHANDLER and her sister.

1859   Acute febrile polyneuritis (Landry paralysis) was
described in two cases of acute ascending paralysis by
German professor, ADOLF KUSSMAUL, and later in the
same year by JEAN BAPTISTE OCTAVE LANDRY, and named
after him.

1859   Jerky movements and echolalia, noted in hysteria and
schizophrenia (Bamberger disease), were described by
German physician, HEINRICH VON BAMBERGER.

1859   AUGUSTA DEJERINE-KLUMPKE born.
An American-born French neurologist who wrote an
important treatise on the neurological features of lead
poisoning, and described lower brachial plexus palsy,
Dejerine-Klumpke paralysis, or waiter's tip (1885).

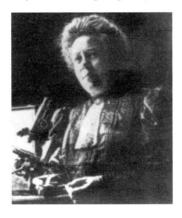

Augusta Dejerine-Klumpke
(1859–1927)

1859 ALBERT KUNTZ born.
A professor of histology at St Louis University, Kentucky who described the gray ramus running from the second thoracic ganglion to the first thoracic nerve (1927).

1860 JOSEPH MERRICK born.
A victim of neurofibromatosis from London who was rescued by FREDERICK TREVES from being a public exhibit, and was later the subject of Treve's biography, *The Elephant Man*.

1860 MATHIEU JABOULAY born.
A French neurosurgeon from Lyons who performed the first sympathetectomy for the relief of vascular disease (1900).

1860 Curare was used in medical practice to relax the muscles in epilepsy.

1860 WILLIAM DOBINSON HALLIBURTON born.
A professor of physiology from King's College, London who wrote The *Essentials of Chemical Physiology* (1892), and was the first to study the chemical composition of cerebrospinal fluid.

1860 THOMA JONNESCO born.
A professor of surgery at Bucharest who described the retro-duodenal fossa (Jonnesco fossa or fold, 1889), and carried out an operation for the removal of the cervical ganglia of the sympathetic trunk (Jonnesco operation).

1860 Catatonia was described and named by KARL L KAHLBAUM of Germany.

1860   The clinical state of nervous exhaustion and asthenia was named 'nervosisme' by Paris physician, JEAN EUGÉNE BOUCHUT.

1860   CHARLES ÉMILE ACHARD born.
A Paris physician who introduced one of the first tests for renal function, described paratyphoid fever, wrote on encephalitis lethargica, and edema in Bright disease.

1860   S HEINRICH FRENKEL born.
A medical superintendent from Switzerland who advocated the use of extensive physiotherapy for neurological disease with his introduction of exercises for tabetic ataxia (1890), and wrote *The Treatment of Tabetic Ataxia by Means of Systematic Exercise*.

1861   The Trousseau sign, an indication for hypocalcemia involving tetanic spasm of the hand on applying sufficient pressure to the arm, was described by ARMAND TROUSSEAU of Paris.

1861   CHARLES GILBERT CHADDOCK born.
An American neurologist who described an extensor plantar response obtained by stroking the skin in the area of the external malleolus in cases of pyramidal tract lesions (Chaddock sign).

1861   The involvement of the Gasserian ganglion of the trigeminal nerve in herpes zoster infection of the face was described by FRIEDRICH VON BÄRENSPRUNG.

1861   ALESSANDRO CODIVILLA born.
An Italian orthopedic surgeon who wrote on tendon transplantation and the redistribution of muscles power around the joints, using this in spastic paralysis.

1861 Cerebral palsy with mental deficiency and muscle weakness in the newborn (spastic diplegia or Little disease), due to a variety of causes such as asphyxia, birth injury and prematurity, was described by WILLIAM LITTLE of London.

1861 Experimental research on the action of the vagus and cervical sympathetic nerves on the heart, respiration, stomach, ear and pupils was carried out by English physiologist, AUGUSTUS VOLNEY WALLER.

1861 WILHELM HENDRIX COX born.
A Dutch bacteriologist who introduced a process of impregnating nerve cells and neuroglia with potassium salts, mercuric chloride and ammonia for histological studies.

1861 SIR HENRY HEAD born.
A London neurologist who mapped the cutaneous areas of the sensory nerve roots related to visceral organs (1893), and published an important work on speech defects, *Aphasia and Kindred Disorders of Speech* (1926).

1861 Meniere syndrome, episodic vertigo, tinnitus and progressive deafness, was described by French otorhinologist, PROSPER MENIERE.

1862 The muscle spindle or the stretch afferent (Ruffini corpuscle) was studied by WILLY KÜHNE, and then later in detail by Italian professor, ANGELO RUFFINI.

1862 ERNEST DUPRÉ born.
A French physician who described a form of psychoneurosis in which the patient makes a conscious effort to control his symptoms (Dupré disease).

1862   A mass of ganglia on the cardiac nerves in the atrial septum (Ludwig ganglion) was described by the eminent German physiologist, KARL FRIEDRICH LUDWIG.

1862   A network of autonomic nerve fibers in the intestinal wall, the Auerbach plexus, was described by German neuropathologist, LEOPOLD AUERBACH.

1862   LOTHAR VON FRANKEL-HOCHWART born.
An Austrian neurologist who described cochlear, vestibular and trigeminal lesions (Frankel-Hochwart disease), seen in early syphilis.

1862   ADOLF WALLENBERG born.
A German neurologist who described Wallenberg syndrome of ipsilateral loss of pain sensations in the face, with contralateral hypoesthesia for pain and temperature of the trunk due to occlusion of the posterior cerebellar artery (1895).

1862   Raynaud disease was described by French physician, MAURICE RAYNAUD of Paris, who presented several cases of intermittent cyanosis on exposure to cold, as local asphyxia of the extremities.

1863   Silver stain to study nerve endings in the muscles was introduced by JULIUS FRIEDRICH COHNHEIM, a German pathologist from Poland.

1863   Paralysis of the vocal cord due to a recurrent laryngeal nerve lesion (Gerhardt syndrome) was studied by Berlin physician, CARL ADOLF CHRISTIAN GERHARDT.

1863 A syndrome of hemiplegia with contralateral paralysis of the oculomotor nerve secondary to a lesion in the cerebral peduncle (Weber syndrome) was described by London physician of German origin, SIR HERMAN WEBER.

1863 SIMON FLEXNER born.
An American bacteriologist and the first director of the Rockefeller Institute who studied *Shigella flexneri* (the causative agent of dysentery, 1900), and prepared antiserum to treat cerebrospinal meningitis (1908).

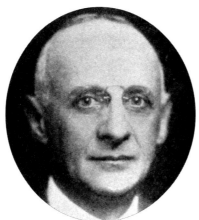

Simon Flexner
(1863–1946)

1863 The lateral nucleus of the 8th nerve was described by German physician, OTTO FRIEDRICH DEITERS, who also discovered astrocytes in nerve tissue in the same year.

1863 GEORGES MARINESCO born.
A neurologist from Bucharest, Romania, who described trophic changes in the skin of the hand in cases of syringomyelia.

1863 The five branches of nerves arising from the sphenopalatine ganglion (Randacio nerves) were described by a professor of anatomy at the University of Palermo, FRANCESCO RANDACIO.

1863 ALBERT ABRAMS born.
A German-born physician in San Francisco who invented spondylotherapy in which he applied pressure to points in the spine as treatment for a variety of illnesses.

1863 German physiologist, ALBERT VON BEZOLD, described the nerve ganglia in the interauricular septum, the Bezold ganglia, and found the accelerator nerve fibers of the heart and their origin in the spinal cord (1862).

1863 Speech impairment, lateral curvature of the spine and swaying of the body with irregular movements (Friedrich ataxia) was described by NIKOLAUS FRIEDRICH, a German physician from Heidelberg. He also wrote a significant treatise on progressive muscular atrophy.

1863 LEO M CRAFTS born.
An American neurologist who described dorsiflexion of the great toe when the anterior surface of the ankle is stroked in cases of pyramidal tract lesions.

1863 WILLIAM GIBSON SPILLER born.
An American neurologist who described arachnoiditis and chronic inflammation of the spine in a patient as 'meningitis circumscripta spinalis', one of the earliest descriptions of this disease.

1864   Cortical areas responsible for specific isolated movements in the body were proposed in an early treatise by British neurologist, JOHN HUGHLINGS JACKSON, who described a unilateral localized form of epilepsy (Jacksonian).

1864   HENRI FRAENKEL born.
A Paris ophthalmologist who described the upward rolling movement of the eye during an attempt to close the eyelids in cases of lower motor neuron paralysis of the facial nerve.

1864   LOUIS FISHER born.
A New York physician who gave his name to the systolic murmur (Fisher murmur) heard in the anterior fontanel of the temporal region in cases of rickets.

1864   ALOIS ALZHEIMER born.
A German psychiatrist who described the most common cause of senile dementia (Alzheimer disease, 1907), after studying the brains of demented and senile patients at autopsy in Munich.

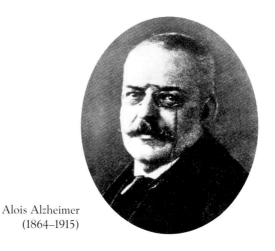

Alois Alzheimer
(1864–1915)

1865   IRA VAN GIESON born.
A New York neuropathologist who devised a histological
staining method for tissues, using alum–hemotoxylin (Van
Gieson stain).

1865   Russian physiologist, ELIE DE CYON, showed that stimulation
of the aortic depressor nerve causes a drop in blood pressure.

1865   NORBERT ORTNER born.
A professor of medicine in Vienna, Austria, who
described paralysis of the left vocal cord due to an
enlarged left atrium in mitral stenosis (Ortner
syndrome).

1865   EGMONT MUNZER born.
A professor of medicine at Prague who described the tract
from the internal geniculate body to the lateral part of the
pons (Munzer tract, 1895).

1865   CHRISTIAN ARCHIBALD HERTER born.
A pathologist in New York who described infantilism
due to chronic intestinal infection (Herter disease, 1908),
published studies on experimental myelitis (1889), and
founded the *Journal of Biological Chemistry* (1905).

1866   Miliary aneurysms were described by ABEL HENRY
BOUCHARD, who associated these with cerebral
hemorrhage.

1866   FRITZ LANGE born.
A German orthopedic surgeon who transplanted biceps
in cases of paralyzed quadriceps, used silk thread to
extend tendons, and wrote on poliomyelitis.

1866 HANS HELD born.
A Prussian professor of anatomy at Leipzig who described decussation of specific acoustic nerve fibers in the lateral fillet (a lemniscus in the trapezoid body) in 1891.

1866 ADOLF MEYER born.
A Swiss-born American psychiatrist and neurologist who proposed the concept of psychobiology which integrated medicine and psychiatry, and sought to explain mental disorders on the basis of maladjustment.

1866 An ethnic classification for the mentally retarded, including a group named Mongolian, giving rise to the term Mongol, was proposed by JOHN LANGDON HAYDON DOWN of England. An important figure in mental care who published a blueprint for treatment and education of the mentally retarded, *Observation of Ethnic Classification of Idiots*.

1866 ALBIN LAMBOTTE born.
A Belgian surgeon who carried out an early craniotomy, created osteosynthesis and surgical instruments for this.

1866 CLAUDIEN PHILLIPE born.
A director of the Pathological Anatomy Laboratory in the Salpêtriére Hospital in Paris who described the septomarginal tract in the sacral region of the spinal cord (1901).

1867 THEODOR FRITSCH, a military surgeon during the Franco-Prussian war, studied soldiers suffering from brain damage, and noted that stimulation of one side of the brain caused the opposite side to twitch.

1867   Eminent English psychiatrist, HENRY MAUDSLEY, maintained that insanity was fundamentally a bodily disease in his *The Physiology and Pathology of the Human Mind*.

1867   EDMUND BIERNACKI born.
A Polish physician in Austria who described analgesia of the ulnar nerve in dementia paralytica and tabes dorsalis (Biernacki syndrome).

1868   Deviation of the eyes, the deviation to the side of the lesion of the cerebral hemisphere, was described by Swiss physician, JEAN LOUIS PREVOST.

1868   Progressive joint damage due to excessive movement range, caused by loss of pain sensation secondary to neuropathy or other neurological disease (Charcot joints), and osteoarthritis attributed to syphilis were described by French neurologist, JEAN MARTIN CHARCOT.

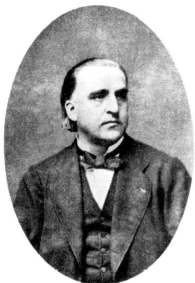

Jean Martin Charcot
(1825 1893)

1868 The fasciculus gracilis of the spinal cord was described
by a neuroanatomist from Zurich in Switzerland,
FRIEDRICH GOLL, who wrote *Minute Anatomy of the Spinal Cord
of Man* (1860).

1868 KORBINIAN BRODMANN born.
A German neuropsychiatrist and pioneer in the localization of
cerebral function who classified the cortical areas of the brain
in numerical terms (Brodmann areas).

1868 A neurogenic reflex arising in the lung and controlling the
rate and depth of respiration via the vagus nerve
(Hering–Breuer reflex) was described by Austrian
psychiatrist, JOSEF BREUER and KARL EWALD HERING.

1868 LUDWIG PICK born.
A professor of pathological anatomy in Berlin who described a
disorder of sphingomyelin (Niemann–Pick disease, 1926), and
scleroderma macroglossia, with German pathologist, OTTO
LUBARSCH.

1868 ALFRED WALTER CAMPBELL born.
An Australian pathologist who wrote *Pathology of
Alcoholic Insanity* (1892), defined the precentral area
of the cerebral cortex (Campbell area, 1905), and carried
out studies related to localization of function in the
cerebral cortex.

1869 Meynert decussation on the tracts of tegmenti within the
spinal canal was described by THEODOR HERMAN MEYNERT,
professor of neurology at Vienna, Austria.

1869 The theory that the tympanic membrane of the ear, on receiving sound, vibrated like a microphone and imparted electrical impulses to the brain, was put forward by WILLIAM RUTHERFORD of King's College, London.

1869 Sensory aphasia was described by British neurologist, HENRY CHARLTON BASTIAN.

1869 LUTHER CROUSE PETER born.
A Philadelphia ophthalmologist who designed an operation for oculomotor paralysis, which involved the transplantation of the tendon of the superior oblique muscle.

1869 JAMES PURVES-STEWART born.
A British neurologist at the Royal National Orthopedic Hospital in London who wrote an important textbook of neurology, *The Diagnosis of Nervous Disease*.

1869 HENRI C J CLAUDE born.
A French neurologist who described ipsilateral oculomotor palsy with contralateral ataxia and hemichorea due to a lesion in the red nucleus (Claude syndrome, 1912).

1869 GEORGE MILLER BEARD, an American physician, established the concept of asthenia and nervous exhaustion.

1869 WILFRED HARRIS born.
A neurologist from London who was the first to perform alcohol injection of the Gasserian ganglion through the foramen ovale for treatment of trigeminal neuralgia, and wrote *Neuritis and Neuralgia* (1926).

1869   HARVEY WILLIAMS CUSHING born.
An Ohio neurosurgeon who made important contributions to the study of the pituitary gland and its tumors, and classified cerebral tumors, gliomas and meningiomas, describing techniques for their removal.

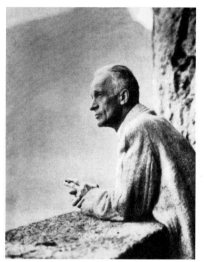

Harvey Williams Cushing
(1869–1939)

1869   A tumor of the meninges (meningioma), usually next to the dura mater, was referred to as an endothelioma by CAMILLO GOLGI, professor of histology at Pavia, Italy.

1870   JAMES STANFIELD COLLIER born.
A London neurologist who described that part of the medial longitudinal bundle within the tegmentum of the midbrain (Collier bundle), and subacute degeneration of the cord.

1870   Irritation of the semicircular canals as a cause of vertigo was shown by German physiologist, FRIEDRICH LEOPOLD GOLTZ. He pioneered work on vestibular disturbances and vertigo, vagal reflex inhibition in relation to the heart, and showed the difference between cortical and subcortical functions.

1870 ROSS GRANVILLE HARRISON born.
An American comparative anatomist who developed the hanging-drop method of tissue culture for growth of nerve fibers from cells outside the organism (1907).

1870 The production of localized motor movements and convulsions in the body due to the stimulation of certain areas of the brain was shown by THEODOR FRITSCH and EDUARD HITZIG of Germany.

1870 Plexiform neurofibroma was described by German surgeon, PAUL VON BRUNS.

1871 Characteristics of childhood persisting into adult life (infantilism) were used by PAUL JOSEPH LORAIN of Paris to denote idiopathic arrest of growth in connection with tuberculosis.

1871 ALFRED FRÖHLICH born.
An Austrian neurologist who described sexual infantilism, obesity secondary to lesions of the hypothalamus (1900), and studied the effects of the pituitary on the autonomic nervous system.

1871 SIR GRAFTON ELLIOT SMITH born.
An Australian neurologist and an authority on brain anatomy and human evolution, who published several important works on evolution, including *Human History*.

1871 KARL LEINER born.
An Austrian pediatrician who described erythroderma desquamation (generalized dermatitis) in children with recurrent local and systemic infection, marked wasting and a deficiency in the central nervous system (Leiner disease).

1871 Sulcus intermedius primus of the cerebral cortex (Jensen sulcus) was described by JULIUS JENSEN, director of the Allenburg Institute of Mental Diseases.

1871 Neuropsychiatrist, KARL FRIEDRICH OTTO WESTPHAL of Berlin, described agoraphobia, demonstrated the absence of knee jerk reflex in tabes dorsalis (1875), and described the third cranial nerve (Edinger–Westphal nucleus, 1887).

1871 LOUIS DUPUYS-DUTEMPS born.
A French ophthalmologist who worked with neurologist RAYMOND CESTAN on pupillary reflexes, and described paradoxical lid retraction present in Bell palsy (Dupuys-Dutemps phenomenon).

1871 CHARLES ALBERT ELSBERG born.
A New York pioneer in neurosurgery who published several papers on olfactory sensation and vision in 1938, and a book on neurosurgery in 1916.

1871 Hammond disease, or athetosis, a failure to maintain a fixed posture due to abnormal involuntary movements, was described by American neurologist, WILLIAM ALEXANDER HAMMOND in his *Diseases of the Nervous System*. He also studied snake venom and arrow poisons, and was a founder of the American Neurological Association.

1872 French neurosurgeon HENRY DURET and JOHANN OTTO LEONHARD HEUBNER of Germany described the distribution of blood vessels within the substance of the brain.

1872 GATIAN DE CLÉRAMBAULT born.
A French psychiatrist who described a state in which the patient believes his mind is controlled by someone else or by external forces (Clérambault–Kandinsky syndrome).

1872 CARL F O WESTPHAL described acute disseminated encephalomyelitis.

1872 WILFRED BATTEN TROTTER born.
An English neurologist who studied the pathology and symptoms of post-head injury status, defined concussion (1924), and described Trotter syndrome (associated with deafness, palatal paralysis and facial neuralgia, 1911).

1872 A rare familial disease, accompanied by progressive involuntary movements, ataxia, and mental deterioration (Huntington chorea/disease) was described by American physician, GEORGE HUNTINGTON.

1872 JAMES SHERREN born.
An English surgeon who studied the consequences of injury to the peripheral nerves in man (1905).

1872 Clinical types of lead palsy, including wrist drop, were described in detail by French neurologist, GUILLAUME B A DUCHENNE.

1872 PERCY THEODORE HERRING born.
A professor of physiology at St Andrew's University in Scotland who showed the spinal origin of cervical sympathetic nerves (1903), and named the Herring bodies in the posterior lobe of the hypophysis.

1873 HENRI DURET of France described the circulation of blood within the brain.

1873 OTFRIED FOERSTER born.
A neurologist from Breslau who advocated intradural division of the posterior nerve roots as treatment for pain.

1873 OTTO LOEWI born.
A German-born American pharmacologist and Nobel laureate (1936) who isolated the first neurotransmitter (1921), showing that a substance liberated from the stimulated vagus nerve ending, when perfused onto a second heart, was capable of slowing the heart rate.

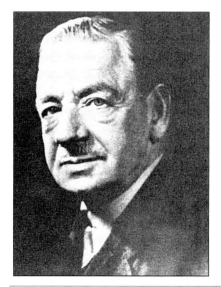

Otto Loewi
(1873–1961)

1874 The Schmidt clefts, found intersegmentally in the medullary sheath of the peripheral nerves, were described by HENRY SCHMIDT, a pathologist at the Charity Hospital in New Orleans.

1874 ARTHUR SCHÜLLER born.
An Austrian physician who first developed skull X-rays for the diagnosis of epilepsy.

1874 OCTAVE CROUZON born.
A French neurologist who carried out important work on hereditary dystrophies, described craniofacial dysostosis and hypertelorism, due to autosomal dominant inheritance (Crouzon disease).

1874 The giant motor cells in the 5th layer of the cerebral cortex, the Betz cells, were described by Russian anatomist, VLADIMIR BETZ.

1874 ALFRED GORDON born.
A neurologist in Philadelphia who described the extensor plantar response produced by squeezing the calf muscles (Gordon reflex) in cases of pyramidal tract lesions.

1874 German neuropsychologist, KARL WERNICKE, described Wernicke encephalopathy, ophthalmoplegia, nystagmus, and ataxia with tremors from thiamin deficiency.

1874 The brain center for olfactory function was studied by Scottish neurologist, SIR DAVID FERRIER.

1874 GEORGES FROIN born.
A French physician who described inflammation of the meninges with obstruction of the spinal subarachnoid space associated with a coagulable state of the cerebrospinal fluid (Froin syndrome, 1903).

1874 Contraction of the abdominal muscles on compression of the testicles (testicular reflex) was described by Swiss surgeon, THEODOR KOCHER.

1874 JOSEPH ERLANGER born.
An American physiologist and Nobel laureate (1944) from the Johns Hopkins Hospital who studied nerve conduction, and proved that the velocity of the impulse was proportional to the diameter of the nerve fiber.

1874 FREDERICK PARKER GAY born.
An American pathologist who studied the cell count in cerebrospinal fluid in poliomyelitis.

1874 ANTONIO EGAZ MONIZ born.
A Portuguese neurologist who introduced a method of radiologically visualizing cerebral circulation by injecting radio-opaque sodium iodide into the carotid artery (1927), and performed the first frontal lobotomy (1935).

1874 ALAN BUCHNER KANAVEL born.
A Kansas surgeon who described the Kanavel sign, a point of maximal tenderness in infections of the tendon sheath and found in the palm, proximal to the base of the little finger.

1874 Application of electrodes to the human cortex to produce contralateral muscle contractions was demonstrated by American physician, ROBERTS BARTHOLOW.

1875 The American Neurological Association was founded.

1875   Evidence for electrical activity in the brain of living animals (electroencephalography) was provided by RICHARD CATON, an English neurologist from Liverpool.

1875   French physicist, GABRIEL JONAS LIPPMAN, invented the capillary electrometer for magnification of minute fluctuations in electrical potential.

1875   FREDERICK TILNEY born.
The father of the New York School of Neurology whose *The Brain from Ape to Man* is considered a classic on modern evolution, and who wrote (with HENRY ALSOP RILEY, 1921) *The form and functions of the central nervous system.*

1875   CECILE VOGT born.
A French neurologist who carried out early work on neuroanatomy of the thalamus, hereditary pseudobulbar palsy, congenital chorea, and also mapped the brain.

1875   SIR HENRY HALLETT DALE born.
A British physician who won the Nobel Prize (1936) for his work on the transmission of nerve impulses, acetylcholine, norepinephrine, and the discovery of histamine.

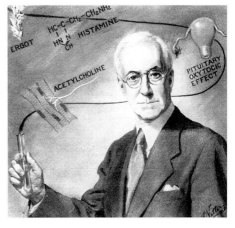

Sir Henry Hallett Dale
(1875–1968)

1876　CONSTANTIN VON ECONOMO born.
An Austrian neurologist who identified and
characterized epidemic encephalitis (1917), and showed
that this was caused by a submicroscopic virus.

1876　Inability to relax muscles after contraction, occurring during
early childhood (Thomsen disease) was described by ERNST
VON LEYDEN and comprehensively by Danish physician,
ASMUS JULIUS THOMSEN.

1876　SIR GORDON MORGAN HOLMES born.
A famous London clinical neurologist who described
primary progressive cerebellar degeneration, and gave an
account of the function of the thalamus and its relationship
to the cerebral cortex (1911), described Holmes–Adie
syndrome of partial iridoplegia (1931), and wrote *The
Spinal Injuries of Warfare* and *The Examination of the Nervous
System*.

1876　Apoplexy caused by cerebral hemorrhage (Broadbent
apoplexy) was described by English neurologist, SIR
WILLIAM HENRY BROADBENT. He proposed Broadbent's
hypothesis for the recovery of motor power of the muscles
in paralysis.

1876　ALEXANDER BITTORF born.
A German pathologist who described the Bittorf sign of pain
in the distribution of the genitofemoral nerve due to lesions of
the testis or ovary.

1876　The Chvostek sign, where the facial muscles go into spasm on
tapping the facial nerve, a diagnostic sign in tetany, was
described by Austrian surgeon, FRANTISEK CHVOSTEK.

1876   ANDRE LATARGET born.
A French professor of anatomy at Lyon who described the anterior gastric nerves used for selective vagotomy.

1876   The pyramidal tract was identified and named by PAUL EMIL FLECHSIG of Leipzig, Germany.

1876   *Localization and Functions of Cerebral Diseases*, an early neurological treatise, was published by JEAN MARTIN CHARCOT of Paris.

1877   The first definite account of myasthenia gravis, caused by a disorder in neuromuscular function due to the presence of antibodies to acetylcholine receptors, was given by English physician, SIR SAMUEL WILKS.

1877   Several vaccines, such as tuberculin, typhoid and rabies, were introduced as shock therapy for syphilis by Austrian psychiatrist, JULIUS WAGNER-JAUREGG, who also investigated the relationship between cretinism and goiter.

1877   Juvenile paresis was associated with congenital syphilis by SIR THOMAS CLOUSTON from Orkney, a superintendent at the Royal Morningside Asylum. He lectured on mental diseases, focused on the mental aspect of adolescence, and published *The Hygiene of the Mind* and *Clinical Lectures on Mental Diseases*.

1877   LOUIS GASTON LABAT born.
A French surgeon in Paris who devised a glass and metal device for locking a needle with a finger hold (Labat syringe), and perfected a method of infiltration of nerves to produce nerve block for anesthesia.

1877 The role of chemicals in the transmission of nerve impulses was suggested by German physiologist, EMIL HEINRICH DUBOIS-REYMOND.

1878 ROBERT BING born.
A French professor of neurology who described the extension of the big toe following stimulation of the dorsum of the foot in cases of pyramidal tract lesions (Bing sign).

1878 CAMILLE BIOT born.
A French physician who described a variant of Cheyne–Stokes respiration seen in medullary compression of the brain, the Biot sign.

1878 The nodes of Ranvier, interruptions in the medullary nerve fiber sheath, were described by LOUIS ANTOINE RANVIER, a neurologist from Paris.

1878 Meralgia parasthetica, affecting the external cutaneous nerve of the thigh and known as Bernhardt disease, was described by German neurologist, MARTIN MAX BERNHARDT.

1878 WILLIAM SMITH GREENFIELD, a London surgeon, described giant cells in Hodgkin disease.

1879 WILLIAM RICHARD GOWERS, the eminent London neurologist, published *Pseudo-hypertrophic Muscular Paralysis*, Gowers disease.

1879 Angioma of the leptomeninges and ipsilateral portwine stain on the face in the region of trigeminal distribution (Sturge–Weber syndrome) was described by English Quaker physician, WILLIAM ALLEN STURGE.

1879   Surgical removal of a brain tumor arising from the dura mater was performed by SIR WILLIAM MACEWEN, professor of surgery at the Glasgow Royal Infirmary in Scotland. In 1885 he performed the earliest recorded successful removal of a spinal tumor.

1879   KEITH LUCAS born.
An English neurophysiologist who described the all-or-none law, that a given stimulus evokes a maximum contraction or no contraction at all in muscles or motor nerve fibers, and wrote *The Conduction of the Nervous Impulse*.

1879   RENÉ LERICHE born.
An surgeon from France who worked on surgery of the vascular system, pain and peripheral nerve injuries..

1879   WALTER SPIELMEYER born.
A German neuropathologist who studied juvenile amaurotic idiocy caused by lipid metabolism disturbance, and wrote an important book on microscopy of the nervous system.

1879   JULES TINEL born.
A French neurologist from Rouen who described tapping over the carpel tunnel causing paraesthesia over the median nerve distribution of the hand in carpel tunnel syndrome (Tinel sign).

1880   ADOLF STÖFFEL born.
A German surgeon who introduced partial peripheral neurectomy for spastic paralysis.

1880 The term 'narcolepsy', referring to recurrent, uncontrollable episodes of sleep, was coined by French neurologist, JEAN BAPTISTE EDOUARD GELINEAU of Paris.

1880 Tuberous sclerosis of the brain, marked by the formation of tumors on the surfaces of the lateral ventricles and sclerotic areas of the brain surface (Bourneville disease), was described by DÉSIRÉ MAGLOIRE BOURNEVILLE of France.

1880 EDWARD ALFRED COCKAYNE born.
An English physician who described dwarfism, microcephaly, retinal atrophy, mental retardation and progressive upper motor neuron dysfunction with autosomal recessive inheritance (Cockayne syndrome).

1880 The sensory tactile nerve endings (Merkel corpuscles) were described by FRIEDRICH SIGMUND MERKEL, professor of anatomy at Göttingen.

1880 ARTHUR C ALPORT born.
A South African physician who described hereditary nephritis with nerve deafness and infrequently a mild platelet defect and cataracts (Alport syndrome).

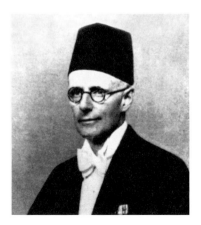

Arthur C Alport
(1880–1959)

1880 The reflex involved in the act of deglutination was described by a German physiologist, KARL HUGO KRÖNECKER.

1880 British ophthalmologist WARREN TAY described amaurotic family idiocy (Tay–Sachs disease) and its ocular manifestations.

1880 The peripheral neuritis of beriberi was described by ERWIN OTTO VON BAELZ.

1880 JEAN ALEXANDER BARRÉ born.
A French professor of neurology at Strasbourg who (with Y. C. LIEOU) described Barré–Lieou syndrome (1928) in which occipital headache, tinnitus, vertigo and facial spasm occur as a result of sympathetic plexus around the spinal column in rheumatoid arthritis of the cervical spine.

1881 The nucleus lateralis of the accessory nerve (Roller nucleus) was described by CHRISTIAN ROLLER, a neuropsychiatrist from Strasbourg in France.

1881 SIGMUND EXNER, professor of physiology at the University of Vienna, described the superficial tangential layer of the cerebral cortex.

1881 WALTER RUDOLF HESS born.
A Swiss physiologist and Nobel Prize winner who worked on the brain as a coordinating organ for the functions of the internal organs and sleep.

1881 *Epilepsy and other Chronic Convulsive Diseases* was published by WILLIAM RICHARD GOWERS, the eminent London neurologist.

1881 The sensory speech center in the posterior third of the gyrus temporalis superior (Wernicke area) was described by German neuropsychiatrist, KARL WERNICKE.

1882 CHARLES FOIX born.
A French neurologist who described the Foix syndrome of ophthalmoplegia due to paralysis of the 3rd, 4th, 5th and 6th cranial nerves, secondary to pathology in the lateral wall of the cavernous sinus (1922).

1882 HEINRICH QUINCKE, a German professor of medicine who spent most of his working career in Switzerland, gave the first description of angioneurotic edema.

1882 Prolongation of the optic tract extending to the 3rd nerve nuclei, the cerebellum and the pons (Stilling root) was described by JAKOB STILLING, professor of ophthalmology in Strasbourg.

1882 ARTHUR JAMES EWINS born.
An English chemist who isolated the neurotransmitter acetylcholine, and whose work led to the development of the antibiotic, sulfapyridine, the first successful treatment for gonorrhea.

1882 Von Recklinghausen disease or neurofibromatosis, multiple tumors of the nerves with café-au-lait spots in the skin, was described by professor of pathology in Königsberg, FRIEDRICH DANIEL VON RECKLINGHAUSEN.

1882 Beriberi was eradicated in the Japanese navy by ADMIRAL KANEHIRO TAKAKI who improved the diet of sailors by adding fresh food to their diet of polished rice.

1882   ROBERT DEBRÉ born.
A French pediatrician who wrote on measles, infectious edematous polyneuritis, muscle hypertrophy, pseudospasm of the pylorus, and sexual infantilism.

1883   Renal osteodystrophy in patients with chronic renal disease (renal rickets) was described by RICHARD CLEMENT LUCAS of Guy's Hospital in London, England.

1883   Noonan syndrome, congenital heart defect, web neck and chest deformity with hypertelorism and mild mental retardation, was observed by O KOBYLINSKI at the Estonian University at Dorpat.

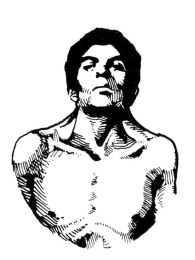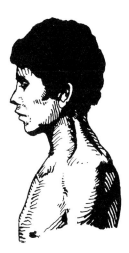

Noonan syndrome

1884   Neural regional anesthesia was performed by injecting cocaine into the inferior dental nerve for dental extraction by American surgeon, WILLIAM HALSTEAD of Johns Hopkins University.

1884   German physician and chemist JOHAN L W THUDICUM, the founder of neurochemistry, published *Chemical Constitution of the Brain*.

1884   The first accurate, clinical localization of brain tumor (which was successfully removed), was made by English neurologist, ALEXANDER HUGHES BENNETT, with RICKMAN JOHN GODLEE.

1884   Landouzy–Dejerine dystrophy, a hereditary form of facio-scapulo-humeral muscular dystrophy transmitted by an autosomal dominant trait, was described by French neurologists, LOUIS THEOPHIL JOSEPH LANDOUZY and JOSEPH JULES DEJERINE.

1884   ROBERT FOSTER KENNEDY born.
A neurologist from Ireland who described shell shock as a form of hysteria, and Kennedy syndrome in *Epilepsy and the Convulsive State*, and wrote on brain tumors and their symptomatology.

1884   Gasserian ganglionectomy was suggested as treatment for trigeminal neuralgia by American surgeon, JAMES EWING MEARS.

1884   HERMANN RORSCHACH born.
A Swiss neuropsychiatrist in Zurich who devised the Rorschach test, a diagnostic procedure in mental disorders and personality tests using standardized ink blots.

1885   The superior vestibular nucleus in the cranial nerve was described by a Russian neurologist, VLADIMIR MIKHAILOVITCH BEKHTEREV. He also described numbness of the spine and a new form of spondylitis.

1885   A specific condition involving peripheral atrophy of the optic nerve (Fuchs atrophy), was described by German oculist, ERNEST FUCHS.

1885   German chemist, PAUL EHRLICH, discovered the blood–brain barrier that prevents many substances dissolved in blood from reaching the brain.

1885   The posterior lateral tract (marginal tract) of the spinal cord, the Lissauer tract, was described by a neurologist from Breslau, HEINRICH LISSAUER.

1885   Ascending and descending branches of the dorsal spinal nerve roots (Nansen fibers) were described by FRIDTJOF NANSEN, Arctic explorer and curator of the Bergen Museum.

1885   Exophthalmos, ptosis and paralysis of the area of the ulnar nerve following injury to the 8th cervical nerve and 1st thoracic root (Dejerine-Klumpke syndrome), was described by AUGUSTA DEJERINE-KLUMPKE of Paris.

1885   SIR FRANCIS MARTIN ROUSE WALSHE born.
A British neurosurgeon who described the symptoms of acroparesthesia and neuritis of the hands caused by pressure from the scalenus anticus muscle in thoracic outlet syndrome (1945).

1885   The rubro-spinal tract (Monakow bundle) was described by Russian neurologist at Zurich, KONSTANTIN VON MONAKOW.

1885   Violent muscular jerks of the shoulders, extremities and face, beginning in childhood with explosive grunting or coprolalia (Tourette syndrome) were described by French neurologist, GEORGES GILLES DE LA TOURETTE.

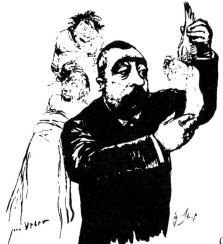

Cartoon of Tourette

1885   The anterior marginal bundle of the cerebellar tract (Löwenthal tract) was described by German physician, WILHELM LÖWENTHAL.

1885   GEORGE ELI BENNETT born.
An American surgeon who worked through polio epidemics and established the first respirator unit for bulbar palsy.

1885   Spinal anesthesia was introduced by American, JAMES LEONARD CORNING.

1885   KARL FRIEDRICH OTTO WESTPHAL of Berlin described a rare form of familial intermittent paralysis in early childhood or adolescence, associated with a low serum potassium (periodic paralysis).

1885   A rabies vaccine was developed from the stored infected brains of animals and used for human inoculation.

1886   WILLIAM JOHN ADIE born.
An English physician who joined the staff of the National Hospital for Nervous Disease and is credited for his original description of narcolepsy.

1886   Chronic lichenoid itching (neurodermatitis or Vidal disease) was described by JEAN BAPTISTE EMILE VIDAL, a dermatologist in Paris.

1886   PAUL SCHILDER born.
A German-born American psychiatrist who observed induration of cerebral substance due to a slow inflammatory reaction (Schilder disease), and identified a subclass where extensive lesions of white matter occurred in both hemispheres.

1886   JEAN-MARTIN CHARCOT and PIERRE MARIE of Paris described an autosomal dominant inherited muscular atrophy due to neurological changes in the spinal cord and nerves (Charcot–Marie–Tooth–Hoffman syndrome).

1886   LEWIS HILL WEED born.
An American neurologist who advanced the theory of cerebrospinal fluid circulation proposed by GUSTAV RETZIUS, and showed that the fluid was absorbed by arachnoid villi.

1886   WALTER EDWARD DANDY born.
An American neurosurgeon who devised a method of
introducing air into cerebral ventricles, treated
trigeminal neuralgia by resection of the trigeminal ganglion
(1934), and described a form of hydrocephalus
(Dandy–Walker syndrome, 1921).

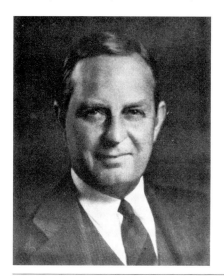

Walter Edward Dandy
(1886–1946)

1886   ARCHIBALD VIVIEN HILL born.
A physiologist from University College London and Nobel
laureate (1922) who measured the heat produced in a
contracting or recovering muscle related to lactic acid
production, and provided an explanation of the transmission
of nerve impulses (1926).

1886   WILLIAM RICHARD GOWERS, a London neurologist, published
one of the most significant works of his era, *Diseases of the
Nervous System*.

1887   The cerebral manifestations and pathology of Tay–Sachs
disease (amaurotic familial idiocy with ocular manifestations)
were pointed out by BERNARD SACHS of New York.

1887 Alfred W Adson born.
An American surgeon and pioneer of neurosurgery who was one of the first to use sympathectomy for treatment of hypertension, and cervical sympathectomy for Raynaud syndrome.

1887 Austrian pathologist, Anton Weichselbaum, isolated the causative organism of cerebrospinal fever (meningitis), *Meningococcus*, from cerebrospinal fluid of patients.

1887 Eduard Gamper born.
An Austrian neurologist who described a reflex seen in children with severe brain damage and occasionally in normal premature babies, due to release of the pons from cortical impulses (Gamper bowing reflex).

1887 Alcohol injection for the treatment of neuralgia was introduced by French physician, Jean Albert Pitres.

1887 Bernhard Dattner born.
A neurologist from the New York University Medical Center who designed a needle for aspirating cerebrospinal fluid, consisting of a fine inner needle within an outer moderate-bore needle for perforating the dura mater.

1887 The infectious nature of acute anterior poliomyelitis was clinically described by Oscar Medin after studying a large outbreak in Sweden.

1887 Gustav Hoffer born.
An otorhinologist from Vienna who described the depressor nerve of the cardiac plexus, a branch of the superior laryngeal nerve.

1887   ROBERT WARTENBERG born.
An American neurologist who described the Wartenberg sign, whereby the little finger is held in ulnar paralysis.

1887   BERNARDO ALBERTO HOUSSAY born.
An Argentine physician and Nobel laureate who contributed to an understanding of feedback mechanisms involved in endocrinology, particularly in relation to insulin, with his work on the pituitary gland.

1887   VITTORIO MARCHI, an anatomist from Florence, Italy described the anterolateral descending tract of the spinal cord (Marchi tract).

1887   DETLEV WULF BRONK born.
An American neurophysiologist who studied the biophysical properties of motor nerve fibers (1927), and recorded the activity of single nerve motor units (1928).

1888   The first successful removal of a brain tumor was carried out by American neurologist and surgeon, WILLIAM WILLIAMS KEEN. In 1907 he published a classic work on thoracic outlet syndrome and the first cervical rib as a cause of pressure symptoms.

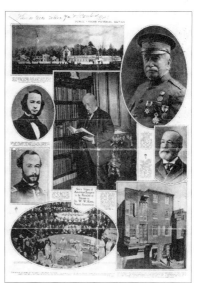

William Williams Keen
(1837–1932)

1888 Pioneering work was carried out on surgical shock by American surgeon and physiologist, GEORGE WASHINGTON CRILE of Cleveland, Ohio. He was one of the first to use blood transfusion and epinephrine in its treatment, and published a monograph on the subject.

1888 An early modern monograph on intracranial tumors was written by BYROM BRAMWELL, a physician to the Edinburgh Royal Infirmary.

1888 A tumor on the spinal cord was removed by the founder of neurosurgery in England, SIR VICTOR ALEXANDER HADEN HORSLEY. He and CLARKE invented apparatus for stereotactic brain stimulation and surgery.

1888 Martinotti cells in the cerebral cortex were described by GIOVANNI MARTINOTTI, professor of anatomy at Bologna, Italy.

1888 WILLIAM RICHARD GOWERS, the eminent London neurologist, described symptoms of fever, vomiting, irritability and headache in cerebrospinal fever.

1888 HERBERT SPENCER GASSER born.
An American physiologist and a director of the Rockefeller Institute for Medical Research who was awarded the Nobel Prize for Physiology or Medicine for his study on the functional differentiation of nerve fibers.

1888 Treatment of neurotic diseases with persuasive therapy or psychotherapy was pioneered by PAUL CHARLES DUBOIS, professor of neurotherapy in Bern.

1888 The cortical visual center was discovered by Swedish pathologist, SALOMON EBERHARD HENSCHEN.

1889 PAUL DIVRY born.
A Belgian neurologist who (with Belgian neuropathologist, Ludo Van Bogaert) described angiomatosis of the skin and cerebral meninges with progressive demyelinization of white matter (Divry–Van Bogaert disease).

1889 LORD EDGAR DOUGLAS ADRIAN born.
A British pioneer in neurophysiology who did valuable work on the activity of the nervous system, later paving the way for the development of the electroencephalogram.

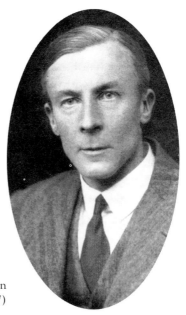

Lord Edgar Douglas Adrian
(1889–1977)

1889 British neurologist, JOHN HUGHLINGS JACKSON, described the temporal lobe as a center for olfactory and gustatory sensations. In 1890 he described a tumor in the right temporosphenoidal area causing olfactory seizures.

1889   An early description of multiple myeloma was given by Bohemian physician, CARL HUGO HUPPERT. His description preceded that of Kahler by a week.

1890   A slow progressive form of hereditary neuritis associated with kyphoscoliosis, arthritis and ocular changes (Dejerine–Sottas syndrome) was described by French neurologists, JULES SOTTAS and JOSEPH JULES DEJERINE.

1890   Frontal lobotomy was performed on four mental patients at a Swiss mental hospital by G BURCKHARD.

1890   French physician, JACQUES ARSENE D'ARSONVAL, showed that it was possible to use electricity to induce anesthesia (electrical anesthesia). He demonstrated that the contraction of muscles brought about by their intrinsic electrical activity could be reversed by applying an external current.

1890   Systematic exercises for tabetic ataxia were introduced by HEINRICH S FRENKEL of the Freihoff Sanitarium in Switzerland, who advocated the use of extensive physiotherapy for neurological disease.

1891   A rare form of familial epilepsy, myoclonus epilepsy, where clonic spasm of a group of muscles occur in paroxysms (Unverricht disease), was described by German physician, HEINRICH UNVERRICHT.

1891   Strümpell disease (polioencephalomyelitis) was described by a German neurologist, ERNST VON STRÜMPELL from Leipzig.

1891 Austrian and German pathologists, HANS CHIARI and JULIUS ARNOLD described Arnold–Chiari syndrome, tongue-like abnormal protrusions of the cerebellum and medulla oblongata.

1891 Osmic acid was used to stain nerve tissue by VITTORIO MARCHI, a histologist and anatomist from Florence, Italy, who also described the anterolateral descending tract of the spinal cord (Marchi tract).

1891 The consequence of removal of the cerebellum in higher mammals was studied by LUIGI LUCIANI. An Italian physician and professor of physiology at Siena, Florence and Rome who described hypotonia, ataxia and weakness seen in cerebellar disease (Luciani triad).

1891 Avellis syndrome, unilateral paralysis of the larynx and soft palate, was described by German otorhinologist, GEORG AVELLIS.

1891 A familial form of progressive spinal muscular atrophy (Werdnig–Hoffman syndrome) was described by Austrian neurologist, GUIDO WERDNIG, with German neurologist, JOHANN HOFFMANN.

1891 A form of degenerative change of the spinal cord associated with pernicious anemia (Dana syndrome) was described independently by CHARLES LOOMES DANA of New York, and JAMES JACKSON PUTNAM of Boston.

1891 WILDER GRAVES PENFIELD born.
An American-born Canadian neurosurgeon whose research at the Montreal Neurological Institute increased understanding of the higher functions of the brain and causes of diseases such as epilepsy.

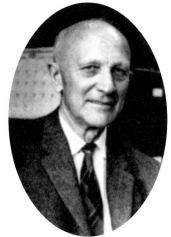

Wilder Graves Penfield
(1891–1976)

1892   SIR VICTOR HADEN HORSLEY and FRANCIS GOTCH localized electrical activity in relation to the different functions of the different compartments of the cerebral cortex.

1892   A form of dementia due to cerebral atrophy of the frontal and temporal lobes (Pick disease) was described as circumscribed cortical atrophy by ARNOLD PICK, a Czech psychiatrist at the University of Prague. He described aperceptive blindness with central atrophy, where the patient cannot fix reflexly on objects (Arnold Pick syndrome).

1892   A form of myotonia which develops in adult life following trauma or infection (Talma disease) was described by SAPE TALMA, a Dutch physician from Utrecht.

1893   The cutaneous areas of the sensory nerve roots related to visceral organs were mapped by SIR HENRY HEAD, a London neurologist.

1893 The islets of the olfactory cells in the hippocampal cortex were described by Spanish anatomist, CAMILLO SANCHEZ CALEJA.

1893 Hereditary cerebellar ataxia, a disease of late childhood involving lack of coordination, was described by PIERRE MARIE of Paris.

1893 British physiologist, JOHN NEWPORT LANGLEY, identified and named the parasympathetic nervous system, postganglionic and preganglionic nerves. In 1894 he and HUGH KERR ANDERSON used the term 'axon reflex' to denote the reflex response of the urinary bladder to nerve stimulation. Langley was also the founder–owner of the *Journal of Physiology.*

1894 Neuritis of the optic nerve accompanied by acute loss of vision, central scotoma and myelitis (Devic neuromyelitis optica) was described by French physician, EUGÈNE DEVIC.

1894 The sensory nature of the muscle spindle was demonstrated by SIR CHARLES SCOTT SHERRINGTON, professor of physiology at Oxford. His demonstrated decerebrate rigidity by transection of the spinal cord through the upper part of the midbrain (1897), and found proprioceptors, highly specialized somatic sensory end organs of the muscles, tendons and joints (1906).

1894 Chromophil granules in the cytoplasm of nerve cells (Nissl bodies) were discovered by Bavarian neurologist, FRANZ NISSL, using an alcohol-based stain for extranuclear RNA in nerve cells (Nissl stain).

1894 THOMAS FITZHUGH born.
An American physician who (with ARTHUR H CURTIS) described pain in the right upper quadrant of the abdomen due to gonococcal peritonitis (Fitzhugh–Curtis syndrome).

1894 An early form of subcortical encephalopathy leading to a classic picture of dementia in the fifth and sixth decade of life (Binswanger disease) was described by a professor of psychiatry at Jena, OTTO LUDWIG BINSWANGER.

1894 WILLIAM RICHARD GOWERS, the eminent London neurologist, coined the term 'fibrositis'.

1894 The association between cardiac abnormalities and Down syndrome was noted by London physician, EDWARD ARCHIBALD GARROD. He was also the first to describe the concept of storage diseases of the nervous system.

1895 Ipsilateral loss of sensation to pain and temperature due to vascular occlusion of the inferior cerebellar artery (posterior inferior cerebellar artery syndrome) was described by ADOLF WALLENBERG of Berlin.

1895 Partial recovery of the facial nerve after suturing it to an accessory nerve was demonstrated by a neurologist at the Westminster Hospital, SIR JAMES PURVES STEWART, and London neurosurgeon, SIR CHARLES BALLANCE.

1895 WALTER FREEMAN born.
An American neurosurgeon who advocated prefrontal lobotomy in cases of specific mental diseases.

1895 EDWARD GEORGE LIDDELL born.
An English neurophysiologist who worked on tendon
reflex activity with Nobel Prize winner, SIR CHARLES
SHERRINGTON in Oxford, and co-wrote *Reflex Activity
of the Spinal Cord*.

1895 Trendelenburg gait, caused by paralysis of the gluteal
muscles, was described by German surgeon, FRIEDRICH
TRENDELENBURG.

1895 Circulatory collapse in cerebrospinal meningitis
(Waterhouse–Friderichsen syndrome) was originally described
by ARTHUR FRANCIS VOELCKER.

1895 Swedish histologist, HAMMARBERG, pioneered architectonics,
the subdivision of the brain into different regions of different
structure.

1895 *Cryptococcus neoformans*, a fungus found in fruit juice that
infects the nervous system, was described by F SANFELICE of
Italy.

1896 NICHOLAS BERNSTEIN born.
A Russian physiologist who developed the concept of
self-regulated motor systems and cybernetics, which arose
from his study of the physiological mechanisms involved
in human locomotion.

1896 JULES FRANÇOIS BABINSKI published a description of an
abnormal extensor plantar response in pyramidal lesions (the
Babinski reflex) in his *Sur le Reflexe Cutane Plantaire dans
Certaines Affections du Systeme Nerveux Central*, and described
the Babinski syndrome, associated with cardioaortic syphilis
and neurosyphilis.

1896
The theory that changes in cerebral circulation were secondary to alterations in general circulation was proposed by British physiologist, SIR LEONARD ERSKINE HILL.

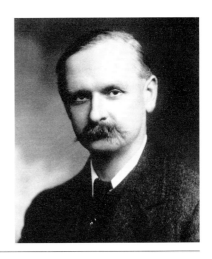

Sir Leonard Erskine Hill
(1866–1952)

1896
JOHAN OTTO LEONHARD HEUBNER of Germany isolated meningococci from cerebrospinal fluid, and described syphilitic endarteritis of cerebral vessels, and an infantile form of idiopathic steatorrhea.

1896
SIR HUGH WILLIAM BELL CAIRNS born.
An Australian neurologist who gave a clear description of hydrocephalus following obstruction of the flow of cerebrospinal fluid secondary to tuberculose meningitis (1949).

1897
CHARLES N ARMSTRONG born.
A British neurologist who successfully treated myxedema with extract of sheep thyroid.

1897
JOHN FRANKLIN ENDERS born.
An American bacteriologist who cultivated the polio virus in human tissue, which led to the development of the polio vaccine.

1897   Muscular rigidity of the body produced by transection of the spinal cord through the upper part of the midbrain was described by SIR CHARLES SCOTT SHERRINGTON of Oxford University, England.

1897   PIOTRE KUZMICH ANOKHIN born.
A Russian psychologist who proposed the concept of a self-regulatory system for the body (feedback mechanism).

1898   YVUNGE ZOTTERMAN born.
A Swedish neurophysiologist who worked with British neurologist EDWARD DOUGLAS ADRIAN on recording and analyzing nerve impulses, and examined the thermal and pain sensations of the skin.

1898   Chemical extraction of the active principle of the suprarenal gland (epinephrine) was performed by American biochemist JOHN JACOB ABEL of Johns Hopkins Medical School.

1898   The first attempt to classify neurons in the spinal and other ganglia was made by ALEXANDER STANISLAVOVITCH DOGIEL, a neurologist and professor of histology at St Petersburg.

1898   The term 'cleidocranial dysostosis' was introduced by a French neurologist, PIERRE MARIE.

1898   The superior nucleus of the vestibular nerve was described by Russian neurologist, VLADIMIR MIKAILOUITCH BEKHTEREV.

1898   French inventor, JACQUES ARSENE D'ARSONVAL, demonstrated that the contraction of muscles brought about by their intrinsic electrical activity could be reversed by applying an external current, suggesting a clinical use for electricity.

1898   HAROLD GEORGE WOLFF born.
A professor of physiology at Cornell University who wrote on gastric function (1943), and jointly published a treatise on pain with STEWART GEORGE WOLFF (1946).

1899   Enlargement of the sella turcica on a skull X-ray in a case of acromegaly was shown by Berlin neurologist, HERMANN OPPENHEIM. In 1900 he described Oppenheim disease, a form of myopathy in infants, amyotonia congenita.

1899   JUDA HIRSCH QUASTEL born.
A British biochemist and a pioneer in biochemical aspects of brain disease, who developed liver function tests for schizophrenia, and worked on the role of glutamic acid in brain metabolism.

1899   The denial of visual disturbance, Anton syndrome, was described by Austrian neurologist, GABRIEL ANTON, who linked brain pathology with psychology in pioneering work on the lack of self perception of deficits in patients with cortical blindness and deafness.

1899   DAME ANNIE JEAN MACNAMARA born.
An Australian physician who discovered that there was more than one strain of the poliomyelitis virus, which paved the way for the development of the Salk vaccine.

1899 FELIX TURYN born.
A Polish physician from Warsaw who described pain in the gluteal region if the great toe is bent in cases of sciatica.

1900 Sympathectomy for relief of pain due to vascular disease was performed by MATHIEU JABOULAY of Paris.

1900 MANFRED JOSHUA SAKEL born.
A French physician who introduced insulin shock in the treatment of schizophrenia.

1900 SIR HENRY HEAD, a London neurologist, and ALFRED W CAMPBELL, studied herpes zoster and established that the disease is an inflammation of the posterior nerve ganglia and roots.

1900 BERNARD J ALPERS born.
An American neurologist who wrote on vertigo, dizziness and clinical neurology, and described progressive cerebral poliodystrophy (Alpers disease).

1901 The descending posteriomedial part of the spinal tract was described by Scottish neurologist, ALEXANDER BRUCE.

1901 DOROTHY H ANDERSEN born.
An American pediatrician and pathologist who described cystic fibrosis of the pancreas (Andersen syndrome).

1901 Extradural caudal injection was introduced independently by JEAN ATHANASE SICARD, a Paris neurologist, and FERNAND CATHELIN, a surgeon from the same city.

1901   DEREK DENNY-BROWN born.
A neurologist from New Zealand who studied the reaction of a single motor neuron (1929), described bronchogenic carcinoma associated with degeneration of the dorsal ganglion cells and myopathy (Denny-Brown syndrome), and designed the cystogram (1933).

1902   The Reed–Sternberg cell, a characteristic cell found in Hodgkin disease, was described by DOROTHY REED of Johns Hopkins Hospital, and was first recognized by Austrian pathologist, KARL VON STERNBERG four years earlier.

1902   The Wiesel paraganglion in the cardiac plexus of the nerves was described by JOSEF WIESEL, professor of medicine at Vienna.

1902   British physician, JOSEPH EVERETT DUTTON, identified the trypanosome in human sleeping sickness.

1902   The symptomatology of frontal lobe lesions was studied in detail by P SCHUSTER of Germany who, with H PINEAS in 1926 studied the grasp reflex in frontal lobe lesions.

1902   Avoidance of shock by nerve block during amputation and observation of blood pressure was advocated by American neurosurgeon, HARVEY WILLIAMS CUSHING of the Johns Hopkins Hospital in Baltimore.

1902   The effect of an electric current on tissues, causing a change in concentration of electrolytes in membranes (Nernst theory), was put forward by German physicists, WALTHER NERNST and E H RIESENFELD.

1903 Bonnier syndrome, vertigo, trigeminal neuralgia and locomotor weakness due to lesions of the vestibular apparatus and 5th nerve nucleus, was described by Paris physician, PIERRE BONNIER.

1903 HALDAN KEFFER HARTLINE born.
An American physiologist from Johns Hopkins Medical School who pioneered neurophysiology of vision, for which he shared the Nobel Prize in Physiology or Medicine.

1903 Marchiafava–Bignami syndrome, a neurological disorder consisting of tremor, convulsions and coma related to alcohol intake, was described by ETTORE MARCHIAFAVA and AMICO BIGNAMI of Italy.

1903 French neurologist, RAYMOND CESTAN and physician, LOUIS J CHENAIS, described ipsilateral paralysis of the vocal cords and soft palate (Cestan–Chenais syndrome).

1903 Basophilic adenomata of the anterior pituitary was described by JAKOB ERDHEIM from Austria.

1903 The presence of blood in cerebrospinal fluid in cases of meningeal hemorrhage was noted by several workers including the French microbiologist, GEORGE WIDAL. Widal and JEAN NAGEOTTE of France also studied the cell elements of cerebrospinal fluid (CSF).

1903 SIR JOHN CAREW ECCLES born.
An Australian neurophysiologist and Nobel laureate (1963) who proposed that synaptic transmission in the nervous system was an electric rather than a chemical phenomenon, and demonstrated control of the nervous system by inhibitory synapses.

1903 Inflammation of the spinal canal (arachnoiditis) was described in a patient as meningitis circumscripta spinalis by WILLIAM GIBSON SPILLER, J H MUSSER and EDWARD MARTIN.

1903 Bulb-type nerve endings were described by St Petersburg neurologist, ALEXANDER STANISLAVOVIC DOGIEL.

1904 CHRISTIAN GEORG SCHMORL noted that the brains of infants dying from jaundice were yellow at autopsy, and found that certain areas of the brain, such as the basal ganglia, were more intensely colored, and he named the syndrome, kernicterus.

1904 Gradenigo syndrome, acute otitis media followed by abducens nerve or internal rectus palsy, was described by GIUSEPPE GRADENIGO, an Italian otorhinologist.

1905 The study of cell structure and layers of specific areas of the brain (cytoarchitronics) was pioneered by Australian pathologist, ALFRED WALTER CAMPBELL. He defined the precentral area of the cerebral cortex (Campbell area).

1905 GUIDO DAGNINI born.
An Italian neurologist who described how percussion of the radial aspect of the back of the hand causes adduction and extension where there is hyperflexia or pyramidal tract lesion (Dagnini reflex).

1905 Nerve impulses of the heart were shown to be dependent on diffusible potassium compounds by WILLIAM HENRY HOWELL, professor of physiology at the Johns Hopkins Hospital in Baltimore.

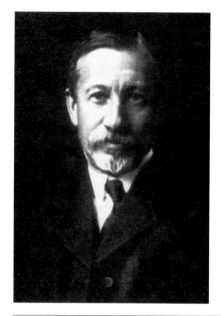

William Henry Howell
(1860–1945)

1905 HANS HELLER born.
A physician from Czechoslovakia who studied water
metabolism (arginine vasotacin) and neurohypophysial
hormones.

1905 Block of thoracic ganglia of the sympathetic chain by
paravertebral injection of drugs (thoracic sympathetic block)
was performed by HUGO SELLHEIM.

1905 The term 'parasympathetic nervous system' was introduced by
JOHN NEWPORT LANGLEY, a neurophysiologist from Newbury,
England, who also coined the terms 'preganglionic' and
'postganglionic'.

1906 Thalamic syndrome, paroxysms of contralateral pain, ataxia
and choreoathetoid movements due to thrombosis or lesions
of the thalamogeniculate artery, was described by JOSEPH JULES
DEJERINE and GUSTAV ROUSSY of Paris.

1906 Recurrent attacks resembling petit mal but not epileptiform in nature (pyknoepilepsy), and a form of relapsing infantile spinal paralysis (Friedmann disease), were described by German physician, MAX FRIEDMANN.

1906 A description of the proprioceptors was given by SIR CHARLES SCOTT SHERRINGTON, an English professor of physiology.

1906 A serum against meningococcal infections was developed by German physician, GEORG JOCHMANN.

1907 A branch of the ramus anterior of the acoustic nerve (Voit nerve) was described by German embryologist and professor of anatomy, MAX VOIT.

1907 The pioneer of spinal analgesia in England, ARTHUR E BAKER of University College Hospital in London, made use of the curves of the vertebral column and introduced hyperbaric solutions of syovaine in 5% glucose.

1907 Alzheimer disease, a form of presenile dementia, was described and studied by German psychiatrist ALOIS ALZHEIMER at the Emil Kraepelin psychiatric clinic in Munich.

1907 HANS SELYE born.
A Canadian physician who carried out important work on hormonal interactions involving the adrenal and pituitary glands and the hypothalamus on osteoblast multiplication, bone formation and blood sugar level.

1907   London neurosurgeon, SIR CHARLES BALLANCE, described chronic subdural hematoma, investigated the etiology of cancer involving protozoa, and (with VICTOR HORSLEY) was the first to successfully remove a spinal tumor.

1907   HORACE WINCHELL MAGOUN born.
An American neuroscientist and pioneer in neuroendocrinology whose early research was on the structure and function of the hypothalamus in relation to sleep, eating and body temperature.

1908   DAVID G COGAN born.
An American neuro-ophthalmologist who described Cogan syndrome of vertigo, tinnitus, progressive bilateral deafness, pain in the eyes and photophobia, blurred vision, and a congenital form of 3rd nerve apraxia.

1908   EDOUARD BRISSAUD and JEAN A SICCARD described facial spasm and contralateral paralysis of the limbs (Brissaud–Siccard syndrome).

1908   Scottish professor of physiology from St Andrew's University, PERCY THEODORE HERRING, described the presence of colloid droplets in the posterior pituitary, showed the spinal origin of cervical sympathetic nerves, and named the Herring bodies in the posterior lobe of the hypophysis.

1908   Neuralgia of the lower half of the face, nasal congestion and rhinorrhea secondary to a lesion in the pterygo-palatine ganglion (pterygopalatine syndrome), was described by GREENFIELD SLUDER of New York.

1908 A stereotactic apparatus for accurate location of electrodes in the brain was produced by SIR VICTOR HADEN HORSLEY, the founder of British neurosurgery.

1908 The first transmission of polio to monkeys, through inoculation of brain tissue filtrate taken from a fatal case of polio, was made by CARL LANDSTEINER and E POPPER.

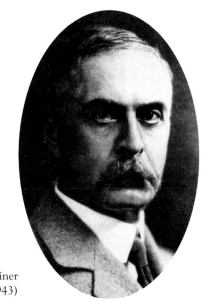

Carl Landsteiner
(1868–1943)

1909 An account of myotonia dystrophica (Curshmann–Batten–Steinert syndrome), frontal baldness, testicular atrophy, dystrophy of sternomastoid muscles and myotonia of lingual muscles, was given by FREDERICK EUSTACE BATTEN of London.

1909 JOHN DAVID SPILLANE born.
A British neurologist who is considered the father of tropical neurology.

1909 German neurologist HANS STEINERT described myotonic dystrophy.

1909 Degeneration of the macula lutea and optic nerve, associated with ataxia, was described by CARL BEHR of Germany and named Behr disease.

1909 RITA LEVI-MONTALCINI born.
An Italian neurologist and Nobel Prize winner (1986) who carried out studies on in vitro nerve growth, and discovered nerve growth factor.

1909 A diagnostic test for meningitis (Brudzinski sign) was described by Polish physician, JOSEF BRUDZINSKI.

1910 The suggestion that secretions of the pancreas depend on a reflex between duodenal mucosa and the vagus nerve was made by Russian Nobel Prize winner, IVAN PETROVICH PAVLOV.

1910 A two-volume work, *Internal Secretions*, which described an eponymous disease of mental deficiency, pituitary change and reduced basal metabolism, was written by Austrian physician, ARTUR BIEDL. He worked on the neural control of the viscera through splanchnic centers, and demonstrated the importance of adrenal glands in internal secretions.

1910 EUGENE BLEULER, a professor of psychiatry in Vienna, described autism in his essay on *Schizophrenias*.

1910 KALMAN PANDY, a Hungarian psychiatrist, devised a method of detecting an increase in globulin in cerebrospinal fluid (CSF).

1910 The electrocardiographic changes of bundle branch block were described by Viennese physician, HANS EPPINGER.

1910   The term 'neurinoma' was introduced by Uruguayan
pathologist, JOSÉ VEROCAY in Prague, to describe a type
of fibroma derived from the endoneurium or the
neurilemma.

1911   An increase in epinephrine output during emotional
stress resulting in palpitations and sweating (Cannon
syndrome) was described by American physiologist,
WALTER BRADFORD CANNON. In 1912 he described the
myenteric reflex which effects the propulsion of food or a
foreign body in the intestines.

1911   Norepinephrine was discovered by GEORGE BARGER and
HENRY DALE of Edinburgh University and the National
Institute for Medical Research. Dale won the Nobel Prize
for his work on the transmission of nerve impulses,
acetylcholine, and norepinephrine.

1911   SIR BERNARD KATZ born.
A German-born British neurophysiologist who worked on
the chemical mechanism of neurotransmission, particularly
acetylcholine, and shared the Nobel Prize for his work on
electrical impulse transmission from nerves to muscles.

1911   Division of the phrenic nerve in the neck to relax the lower
lobe of the lung as treatment in tuberculosis was suggested
by STUERTZ of Cologne.

1911   The first accurate description of the chemical content of
cerebrospinal fluid was given by French neurologist,
WILLIAM MESTREZAT.

1911   Bárány syndrome, described by ROBERT BÁRÁNY in 1918, was first noted by ALFRED BING as cystic serous meningitis of the posterior fossa.

1912   The vascularity of malignant gliomas was shown by English physician, HOWARD HENRY TOOTH. He described the peroneal form of progressive muscular dystrophy (Charcot–Marie–Tooth–Hoffmann syndrome, 1886).

1912   Hepatolenticular degeneration due to abnormality in copper metabolism (Wilson disease) was described by British neurologist, SAMUEL ALEXANDER KINNIER WILSON.

1912   The importance of the unmyelinated nerve fibers in dorsal roots was recognized by Chicago neurologist, STEPHEN WALTER RANSON of Rush Medical College. In 1920 he described neural connections in the hypothalamus.

1912   A theory to explain electrical properties of muscle was proposed by German professor of physiology at Halle, JULIUS BERNSTEIN.

1912   German physician ALFRED HAUPTMANN introduced phenobarbital for treatment of epilepsy.

1912   Ipsilateral paralysis of the 3rd and 4th nerves with contralateral hemianesthesia due to compression of the arterial supply to the inferior nucleus ruber by mesencephalic lesions (Claude syndrome) was described by French neurologist, HENRI C J CLAUDE.

1912   Regulation of temperature was one of the first functions of the hypothalamus discovered by V R ISENSCHMIDT and LUDOLPH VON KREHL.

1912 The findings of Austrian chemist, RICHARD ADOLF ZSIGMONDY, aided analysis of proteins in cerebrospinal fluid (CSF).

1912 TORALD HERMANN SOLLMANN and EDGAR DEWIGHT BROWN of Minnesota described the carotid sinus depressor reflex.

1913 The concept of representing the electrical forces of the heart by recording the vector forces from the surface of the body (vectorcardiography) was proposed by Dutch physiologist, WILLEM EINTHOVEN.

1913 The Lange test for cerebrospinal fluid (CSF), using gold chloride to detect various forms of cerebrospinal syphilis, was devised by CARL FRIEDRICH AUGUST LANGE of Berlin.

1913 ROGER WOLCOTT SPERRY born.
An American neuroscientist who helped establish the way in which nerve cells are wired into the central nervous system and pioneered split-brain experiments.

1913 An early case history for Simmonds disease, hypopituitarism resulting from atrophy of the anterior pituitary lobe, was published by LEON KONRAD GLINSKI of Poland.

1913 STEPHEN WILLIAM KUFFLER born.
An American neurobiologist, born in Hungary, who studied mechanisms of synaptic transmission, retinal physiology, and electrophysiology of glial cells.

1913 A string galvanometer to record the electrical activity of the brain was introduced by Russian physiologist, PRAVDICH NEMINSKY.

1913 Berlin neurologist, HERMAN OPPENHEIM, successfully removed a pineal tumor, with Berlin surgeon, FEDOR KRAUSE.

1913 GEOFFREY W HARRIS born.
A British physician who studied pituitary secretions and their interaction with the brain, and showed the brain is a target organ for ovarian hormones.

1914 WILHELM GENNERICH, a German dermatologist and naval surgeon, introduced treatment of neurosyphilis by intraspinal injections of arsphenamine, and designed a special device for forcing the salvarsanized cerebrospinal fluid into the brain.

1914 Sensory aphasic syndrome accompanied by apraxia and alexia, in lesions of the left parietal lobe, was described by French neurologist, JOSEPH JULES DEJERINE, a pioneer of localization of function in the brain.

1914 Lipoidosis with anemia, mental retardation, retinal degeneration, hepatosplenomegaly and skin pigmentation (Niemann–Pick disease) was described by ALBERT NIEMANN of Berlin.

1914 SIR ALLAN LLOYD HODGKIN born.
A British physiologist who conducted research into nerve impulses in collaboration with SIR ANDREW HUXLEY, with whom he won a Nobel Prize (1963), and described the mechanism by which nerves conduct electrical impulses.

1914 English physiologist, ARTHUR FRANCIS BAINBRIDGE, discovered that cardiac inhibition produced vagal tone, and that accelerator nerves caused cardiac excitation.

1914 The pathway of cerebrospinal fluid was studied by American anatomist, LEWIS HILL WEED.

1915 THOMAS HUCKLE WELLER born.
An American virologist from Michigan and Nobel laureate (1954) who worked on *Schistosoma* and poliomyelitis cell cultivation, and on chickenpox and shingles viruses.

1916 The nature and origin of connective tissue was explained by French neurologist, JEAN NAGEOTTE. He was professor of histology at the College of France, and worked on nerve grafting and the myelin sheath.

1916 An acute ascending form of demyelinating motor neuropathy (Guillain–Barré syndrome) was described by French neurologists, GEORGES GUILLAIN, JEAN ALEXANDER BARRÉ and STROHL.

1916 Unilateral paralysis of the 9th, 10th, 11th and 12th cranial nerves following lesions in the retroparotid space (Villaret syndrome) was described by MAURICE VILLARET of Paris.

1916 A block in the flow of cerebrospinal fluid during lumbar puncture, by applying pressure on the jugular vein (Queckenstedt test), was developed by German physician, HANS HEINRICH QUECKENSTEDT.

1916 FREDERICK CHAPMAN ROBBINS born.
An Alabama physiologist, pediatrician and Nobel laureate (1954) who succeeded in cultivating the poliomyelitis virus, an important step in the development of polio vaccine.

1916   A modern method of trephining the skull for inflammation of the brain was introduced by American surgeon, HARRIS PEYTON MOSHER.

1917   SIR ANDREW FIELDING HUXLEY born.
An English neurophysiologist who provided a physico-chemical explanation for conduction of impulses in nerve fibers, and worked on muscle contraction and relaxation, proposing the sliding filament theory.

1917   A hereditary disease due to a disturbance of mucopolysaccharide metabolism (gargoylism) was described in two brothers by Canadian professor of medicine, CHARLES HUNTER and Austrian pediatrician GERTRUD HURLER (Hunter–Hurler syndrome).

1917   Inattention to objects in one half of the visual field with inability to recognize these objects (Riddoch syndrome) was described by a neurologist from Scotland, GEORGE RIDDOCH.

1917   JEAN ATHANASE SICARD, a Paris neurologist, and French otorhinologist, FRÉDÉRIC JUSTIN COLLET, described palsy of the 9th, 10th, 11th, and 12th cranial nerve as a result of fracture of the posterior cranial fossa (Collet–Sicard syndrome).

1917   The first description of epidemic encephalitis lethargica, a month before ECONOMO'S description, was given by French physician, JEAN RENÈ CRUCHET.

1917 New York neurologist, JAMES RAMSAY HUNT, described a rare form of Parkinsonism due to degeneration of globus pallidus, occurring before the third decade, with facial paralysis, painful ears, vesicular eruption of the oropharynx due to herpes zoster and infection of the geniculate ganglion (Ramsay Hunt syndrome).

1918 A method of introducing air into the ventricles of the brain to visualize it on X-rays was devised by an American neurosurgeon at Johns Hopkins Hospital, WALTER EDWARD DANDY.

1919 London neurosurgeon, SIR CHARLES BALLANCE, published *Essays on the Surgery of the Temporal Bone*.

1919 Neuroglia were differentiated into microglia and oligodendroglia using silver stain by Spanish histologist, PIO DEL RIO HORTEGA of the National Institute for Cancer in Madrid.

1919 H WORSTER, C DROUGHT and A M KENNEDY described death due to circulatory disturbance and neural damage resulting from fulminating meningococcal septicemia.

1919 SIR GODFREY NEWBOLD HOUNSFIELD born.
An English engineer who invented the CAT (computerized tomography) scanner, and shared the Nobel Prize with ALLAN CORMACK of Tufts University in Boston (1979) for his work.

1920 Athetosis, emotional lability and rhythmic oscillation of the limbs due to a lesion in the corpus striatum (Vogt syndrome) were described by French physician CÉCILE VOGT and German neurologist, OSKAR VOGT.

1920 Synaptic transmission was suggested to be more an electrical phenomenon than a chemical mechanism by SIR JOHN CAREW ECCLES, an Australian neurophysiologist.

1920 Puncture of the cisterna magna to obtain a sample of cerebrospinal fluid for diagnostic purposes (occipital puncture) was carried out by Boston neurologist, JAMES BOURNE AYER.

1920 Internuclear ophthalmoplegia in disseminated sclerosis (Lhermitte syndrome) was described by French neurologist, JACQUES JEAN LHERMITTE.

1920 A syndrome of dementia accompanied by pyramidal and extrapyramidal signs which usually occur after middle age (Creutzfeldt–Jakob disease) was originally described by HANS GERHARD CREUTZFELDT and ALFONS MARIA JAKOB.

1920 WILFRED HARRIS, a neurologist at St Mary's Hospital, performed alcohol injection of the Gasserian ganglion through the foramen ovale for treatment of trigeminal neuralgia.

1920 *The Journal of Neurology and Psychopathology* was founded by British–American neurologist, SAMUEL ALEXANDER KINNIER WILSON of the National Hospital, Queen's Square, London.

1920 Neural connections between the hypothalamus and the pituitary were demonstrated by American neuroanatomist, STEPHEN WALTER RANSON of Rush Medical College.

1921 Optic atrophy, ophthalmoplegia and trigeminal neuralgia caused by a lesion in the petrosphenoid space (Jacod triad) was described by French neurologist, MAURICE JACOD.

1921 German-born American pharmacologist and physiologist, OTTO LOEWI of Strasburg, demonstrated that a substance liberated from the stimulated vagus nerve ending, when perfused on to a second heart, was capable of slowing the rate of heart beat.

1921 The first description of grasp reflex, was given by Spanish neurologist, JOSÉ ANTONIO ROVIRALTA BARRAQUER of Barcelona.

1921 Ergotamine was isolated from the ergot fungus, *Claviceps purpurea*, by ARTHUR STROLL, and introduced as treatment in migraine and obstetrics.

1921 Encephalitis lethargica as a cause of Parkinsonism was demonstrated by French neurologist, ACHILLE ALEXANDER SOUQUES.

1921 Failure or obstruction of the foramen of Luschka and Magendie giving rise to hydrocephalus (Dandy–Walker syndrome) was first described by American neurosurgeon, WALTER EDWARD DANDY.

1922 STANLEY COHEN born.
An American neurologist and Nobel Prize winner (1986) who discovered nerve growth factors from *in vitro* tissue culture.

1922 Cavernous sinus syndrome, consisting of paralysis of the 3rd, 4th, 5th and 6th cranial nerves as a result of thrombosis of the cavernous sinus with involvement of its lateral wall, was described by Parisian neurologist, CHARLES FOIX.

1922 Sturge–Weber syndrome, right-sided congenital hemiplegia, accompanied by left-side brain lesions, was described by FREDERICK PARKES WEBER of Temple University, Philadelphia.

1923 The uncommon psychological disorder whereby the patient believes that familiar persons have been replaced by impostors (Capgras syndrome) was described by French psychologist, JEAN MARIE JOSEPH CAPGRAS.

1923 DANIEL CARLETON GAJDUSEK born. An American neurologist and Nobel Prize winner (1976) who worked on the causal agents in degenerative neurological disorders.

1924 Three types of nerve fibers, A, B and C, were described by Nobel laureates (1944), JOSEPH ERLANGER and HERBERT SPENCER GASSER.

1924 The first description of the alpha rhythm in an electroencephalogram (Berger rhythm) was given by German neuropsychiatrist, JOHANNES BERGER.

1924 Austrian pathologist, HEINRICH EWALD HERING, demonstrated the function and structure of the carotid nerve and the reflex effect of pressure in the carotid sinus.

1925 An improved method of encephalography was developed by
LEO MAX DAVIDOFF, a New York neurosurgeon, with
CORNELIUS D DYKE, a radiologist.

1926 DAVID HUNTER HUBEL born.
A Canadian-born American neurophysiologist who studied
cortical perception of visual stimulus, for which he shared the
Nobel Prize for Physiology or Medicine (1981) with ROGER
WALCOTT SPERRY.

1926 Cavernous sinus thrombophlebitis in relation to septicemia
was described by American neurologist, WELLS PHILLIPS
EAGLETON.

1926 NORMAN GESCHWIND born.
He was James Jackson Putnam professor of neurology at
Harvard Medical School and the founder of behavioral
neurology.

1926 *Aphasia and Kindred Disorders of Speech* was published by SIR
HENRY HEAD, a neurologist at the London Hospital and an
expert in speech disorders.

1927 Conclusive proof that the thyroid depended on the
stimulating action of the anterior pituitary was given by PHILIP
EDWARD SMITH of California.

1927 Nobel laureate, ANTONIO EGAZ MONIZ from Portugal,
introduced the method of radiologically visualizing the
cerebral circulation by injecting radio-opaque sodium iodide
into the carotid artery (cerebral angiography).

1929 The suggestion that neurosis is a defect or failure in adjustment to the social environment and arises as a failure to defend the ego was made by Viennese psychologist, ALFRED ADLER.

1929 Reaction of a single motor neuron following its activation by a stimulus was demonstrated by DEREK DENNY-BROWN, a New Zealand-born neurologist at Oxford. He also described bronchogenic carcinoma associated with degeneration of the dorsal ganglion cells and myopathy (Denny-Brown syndrome).

1929 Morquio syndrome, an autosomal recessive disease leading to dwarfism, waddle gait and deafness, but not mental retardation, was described by Uruguayan pediatrician from Montevideo, LUIS MORQUIO.

1930 German dermatologist, KARL THEODORE FAHR, described intracerebral calcification of the small vessels of the deep cortex and lenticular and dentate nuclei (Fahr disease).

1930 Cysticercosis as a cause of epilepsy was identified by a group of British army doctors led by W P MACARTHUR.

1930 Vascular compression as a cause of trigeminal neuralgia was suggested by Baltimore neurosurgeon, WALTER EDWARD DANDY, who later performed partial resection of the sensory root of the trigeminal ganglion.

1930 American biochemist, HARRIET ISABEL EDGEWORTH published a paper on the beneficial effects of ephedrine in myasthenia gravis.

1931 A procedure for direct visualization of the spinal canal through lumbar puncture (myeloscopy) was pioneered by M D BURMAN of America.

1931 American pathologist, MYRTELLE MAY CANAVAN observed a form of familial degenerative disease of the white matter of the central nervous system in Jewish families (Canavan disease).

1932 The first studies on the effect of unilateral lobectomy on patients were performed independently by Canadian neurosurgeon, WILDER GRAVES PENFIELD, and J EVANS, W C GERMAN and J C FOX. PENFIELD'S research at the Montreal Neurological Institute increased understanding of the higher functions of the brain and causes of diseases such as epilepsy.

1932 The study of the biophysical properties of motor nerve fibers was refined by British pioneer in neurophysiology EDGAR DOUGLAS ADRIAN and New York neurophysiologist, DETLEF WULF BRONK, paving the way for development of the electroencephalogram.

1932 Superior sulcus tumor of the apex of the lung, causing pressure on the chest wall, intercostal nerves and brachial plexus (Pancoast tumor) was described by American radiologist, HENRY KHUNRATH PANCOAST of Philadelphia.

1932 SOLOMON ALBERT HYMEN of the Beth David Hospital in New York gave a description of an artificial pacemaker in his experiments on cardiac resuscitation of animals.

1932 A comprehensive work, *Reflex Activity of the Spinal Cord* was published by SIR CHARLES SCOTT SHERRINGTON, an English professor of physiology.

1932 Nerve grafting for facial palsy was introduced by English neurosurgeon, SIR CHARLES ALFRED BALLANCE.

1933 An accurate description of the nerve supply related to uterine pain was given by J G P CLELAND, who employed a series of paravertebral and low caudal blocks in obstetrics.

1933 American pathologist JAMES ROBERTSON DAWSON JR described subacute encephalitis.

1933 Greenfield disease, a fatal familial condition characterized by progressive loss of motor power with seizures, blindness, nystagmus and mental deterioration in children, was described by London neuropathologist, JOSEPH GODWIN GREENFIELD.

1933 Additional features of oral, parotid and skin changes in Sjögren syndrome (keratoconjunctivitis sicca and xerostomia, enlarged parotid gland with polyarthritis) were noted by HENRIK SAMUEL CONRAD SJÖGREN, a Scandinavian neurologist.

1933 The first successful modern surgical technique for treatment of an intracranial aneurysm in the internal carotid artery was that of NORMAN MCOMISH DOTT of Edinburgh.

1933 The causative virus of St Louis encephalitis was isolated by St Louis physicians, R N MACKENFUSS, CHARLES ARMSTRONG and HOWARD M MCCORDOCK.

1934 Inflammation of the temporal and other cranial arteries (temporal arteritis) was described by American physicians, BAYARD TAYLOR HORTON, T B MAGATH and GEORGE ELGIE BROEN.

1934 Norwegian pediatrician IVAR ABSJORN FØLLING described phenylketonuria, the first hereditary metabolic disorder responsible for mental retardation.

1934 British neurologist, MARY BROADFOOT WALKER, introduced the first effective treatment for myasthenia gravis, physostigmine.

1934 American bacteriologists ALBERT BRUCE SABIN and ARTHUR M WRIGHT isolated the herpes simiae virus (B virus) from the brain of a lab worker who died after being bitten by an infected monkey.

1934 Partial resection of the sensory root of the trigeminal ganglion as treatment of trigeminal neuralgia, was performed by WALTER EDWARD DANDY, an American neurosurgeon from Johns Hopkins Hospital.

1934 RENE LERICHE and R FONTAINE used stellate ganglion block, or cervico-sympathetic thoracic block.

1935 The National Foundation for Infantile Paralysis, the first center in the world for research into polio, was established in America.

1935 ANTONIO EGAZ MONIZ and ALMEIDA LIMA, from Portugal, excised the frontal lobe as treatment in a psychiatric patient (the first frontal lobotomy).

1936 In studies on the treatment of pain relief, British neurologist W RITCHIE RUSSELL used intraspinal alcohol injections in cases of terminal cancer.

1936 G H MONRAD–KROHN recognized the role of flicker mechanisms in precipitating epileptic fits, which led to a significant reduction in their numbers.

1936 J A BARGEN and coworkers described autonomic diabetic neuropathy causing diarrhea.

1936 ALFRED BLALOCK of Baltimore performed the first successful thymectomy for myasthenia gravis.

1936 W R JORDAN described neuropathic arthropathy, or Charcot joints, as a complication of diabetes.

1937 Electrically-induced convulsions were given to mental patients by LUCIO BINI and UGO CERLETTI in Italy.

1937 Insulin shock treatment was used for schizophrenia by French physician, MANFRED JOSHUA SACKEL.

1937 An extract of Bulgarian belladonna (deadly nightshade) was introduced as a treatment for post-encephalitic Parkinsonism in England by F J NEWAHL and C C FENWICK.

1938 SOLOMON HALBERT SNYDER born.
An American psychiatrist who investigated the biochemistry of nervous tissue and researched catecholamines from different areas of the brain.

1938 *Physiology of the Nervous System*, published by JOHN FARQUHAR FULTON from Yale University, contains the most comprehensive bibliography and author index on the subject.

1938 Exophthalmic ophthalmoplegia or malignant exophthalmos, was described as a separate entity from Graves exophthalmos by the British neurologist, WALTER RUSSEL BRAIN.

1938 Increased maternal age as a cause of mongolism or Down syndrome was noted by British geneticist, LIONEL SHARPLES PENROSE. He also studied schizophrenia, and carried out a major survey of the causes of mental illness.

1938 Diphenylhydrantoin was introduced as treatment for epilepsy by American neurologists, HIRAM HOUSTON MERRIT of New York and TRACY JACKSON PUTNAM of Boston.

1938 W FELDBERG and C H KELLAWAY introduced the term 'slow reacting substance' for a material obtained from cobra venom and capable of contracting smooth muscle.

1939 English physician, HENRY STANLEY BANKS, used sulfonamide for treating meningococcal meningitis.

1939 A standardized form of curare, Incocostrin, was produced.

1939 An operation to restore the function of the vocal cords was described by American surgeon in Seattle, BRIAN THAXTON KING, and New York otorhinologist, JOSEPH DOMINIC KELLY.

1939 Refsum syndrome, a congenital condition consisting of retinitis pigmentosa, deafness, ataxia and peripheral neuropathy, was described by F THIEBAUT of Paris.

1941 The somatic symptoms of effort syndrome, or soldier's heart, were attributed to psychoneurosis arising from fear by the English cardiologist, PAUL HAMILTON WOOD.

1942 The occurrence of shock in burns and trauma was investigated by American physician, SANFORD M ROSENTHAL.

1942 Shock due to crush injury was demonstrated on an experimental basis by Baltimore surgeon, GEORGE WALTON DUNCAN.

1942 Hungarian scientist and Nobel laureate (1937), ALBERT SZENT-GYÖRGYI, demonstrated the action of the proteins actin and myosin (actomyosin) in bringing about muscle contraction.

1942 H D ADAMS and L V HANDS of Boston did the first successful electrical defibrillation in a human.

1943 BYRON POLK STOOKY described brachial neuritis due to lateral herniation of the cervical intervertebral disc.

1943 American physician, ROY RICHARD GRINKER, studied athetosis arising out of basal ganglionic lesions of the brain.

1943 Sectioning of the supradiaphragmatic vagus nerves as treatment for duodenal ulcers was performed by a Chicago surgeons, LESTER REYNOLD DRAGSTEDT and FREDERICK MITCHUM OWENS.

1944   One of the first units to treat and rehabilitate spinal injuries in England, Stoke Mandeville Hospital, was founded by SIR LUDWIG GUTTMAN.

1944   Intrathecal administration of penicillin in treatment of pneumococcal meningitis was introduced by British neurologist, SIR HUGH BELL CAIRNS and colleagues.

1946   Swedish pharmacologist, Nobel laureate (1970), and pioneer in neurotransmission, ULF SVANTE VON EULER observed raised levels of catecholamines in patients with pheochromocytoma, isolated and studied norepinephrine, and discovered prostaglandins.

1946   British neurologist, SAMUEL ALEXANDER KINNIER WILSON, described a clinical syndrome of basal ganglia lesions associated with paralysis agitans and athetosis.

1947   The use of antihistamines to inhibit the reaction of the autonomic nervous system to physical stress in surgery was investigated by French surgeon, H LABORIT of the Military Hospital in Paris.

1947   Stereotaxic surgery was first used as a treatment for Parkinson disease, to produce discrete lesions in the basal ganglia, by ERNEST ADOLF SPIEGEL, H T WYCIS, M MARKS and A J LEE of New York.

1947   GEORGE EUGENE MOORE introduced fluorescein, a radioisotope, for diagnostic neuroradiology.

1947 An American pioneer in neurosurgery, I CAFFEY ADSON, recommended the division of the scelenus anterior muscle for relief from symptoms of cervical rib syndrome.

1947 In his book, *Hearing*, American physiologist GEORG VON BEKESY, provided a modern study on the mechanism of the ear, and analyzed the manner in which it transmits sound to the brain.

1948 The American Academy of Neurology was founded by ABE BERT BAKER, professor of neurology at the University of Minnesota.

1948 A scientific work on stress, linking it to biological and pathological consequences in man, was produced by HANS SELYE, a Canadian physician of Austrian origin.

1949 Nobel laureate (1954) JOHN FRANKLIN ENDERS, FREDERICK ROBBINS and THOMAS HUCKLE WELLER successfully cultivated a strain of polio virus in human non-nervous tissues.

1949 English pharmacologists WILLIAM PATON and ELEANOR ZAIMUS developed dexamethonium bromide as a ganglion blocking agent.

1949 British neurologist, SIR HUGH CAIRNS, was the first to describe hydrocephalus following obstruction of the flow of cerebrospinal fluid secondary to tuberculose meningitis.

1949 KENDALL BROOKS CORBIN introduced artane, or benzhexol, for treatment of Parkinson disease.

1949 PAUL FURBRINGER born.
A German physician who demonstrated the diagnostic value of spinal tap, and described the Furbringer sign, in which a needle inserted into a subphrenic abscess moved with respiration.

1949 Short-acting muscle relaxants were developed by Nobel laureate (1957) DANIEL BOVET, an Italian pharmacologist (who also prepared antihistamines) and used clinically two years later in Italy and Sweden.

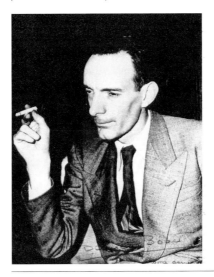

Daniel Bovet
(1907–1992)

1950 CLAUDE SCHAFER BECK, a pioneer in open-heart massage, used the electrical countershock method and direct cardiac massage to the exposed heart to stop intraoperative ventricular fibrillation.

1950 Ataxia, retinitis pigmentosa, and abetalipoproteinemia (Bassen–Kornzweig syndrome) was described by Canadian-born American physician, FRANK ALBERT BASSEN, and New York ophthalmologist, ABRAHAM LEON KORNZWEIG.

1951   A *History of Neurological Surgery*, edited by American neurosurgeon A EARL WALKER of Johns Hopkins Hospital in Baltimore, was published.

1951   British psychiatrist and neuropathologist, ARCHIBALD DENIS LEIGH, described subacute necrotizing encephalomyelopathy (Leigh disease).

1951   Occlusion of the anterior spinal artery resulting in complex neurological signs was described as anterior spinal artery syndrome by KARL BECK of Germany.

1951   O VON DARDEL and S THESLEFF of Sweden used choline esters of succinic acid or suxamethonium for muscle relaxation.

1952   American virologist and Nobel laureate (1956), JONAS EDWARD SALK, developed a killed vaccine against acute poliomyelitis.

1953   The term 'neuroleptic' was applied to certain groups of drugs used in treatment of psychoses by J DELAY, P DENICKER and Y TARDIEU.

1953   The Apgar score was developed by VIRGINIA APGAR of Columbia University, based on observations made of the newborn immediately after birth, and is predictive of the motor and metal development of the child.

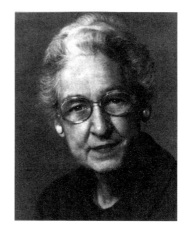

Virginia Apgar (1890–1974)

1953 British neurologist, MACDONALD CRITCHLEY, published his classic book *The Parietal Lobe*. He is considered a founder of neuropsychology and wrote extensively on cognitive function.

1954 Icelandic pathologist, BJORN SIGURDSSON, introduced the concept of slow viral infections.

1954 Menkes syndrome, an inborn error of leucine and isoleucine metabolism leading to mental deficiency, was described by American pediatrician, JOHN H MENKES.

1955 Abdominal decompression as a method of pain relief in labor was introduced by South African gynecologist, O S HEYNS. He applied negative pressure via a shell (Heyns bag) which could be controlled by the patient.

1955 HOUSTON HIRAM MERRIT, professor of neurology at the College of Physicians and Surgeons, Columbia University, published the first modern textbook on neurology. He was the driving force behind the establishment of the National Institute of Neurological Diseases and Blindness in the National Institutes of Health at Bethesda.

1956 A myasthenia-like reaction associated with small-cell carcinoma of the bronchus (Eaton–Lambert syndrome) was described by American neurologists, EDWARD H LAMBERT and LEALDES MCKENDREE EATON at the Mayo Clinic in Rochester.

1956 External ophthalmoplegia, ataxia and areflexia due to a vascular cause (Miller Fisher syndrome) were described by American neurologist, MILLER FISHER.

1957 American virologists, DANIEL CARLETON GAJDUSEK and VINCENT ZIGAS, described kuru amongst the cannibal Fore tribe of Papua New Guinea but were unable to identify its cause. It was later shown to be a form of spongiform encephalopathy. Gajdusek was awarded the Nobel Prize for work on the causal agents in degenerative neurological disorders.

1957 Myoclonic and akinetic seizures in children with a petit mal type of EEG (Lennox–Gastaut syndrome) were first described by French neurologist, HENRI GASTAUT.

1957 The World Federation of Neurology was founded by leading Belgian neurologist and neuropathologist, LUDO VAN BOGAERT, who was its first president.

1958 WILLIAMS and SPENCER used hypothermia to treat patients who sustained neurological damage following cardiac arrest.

1959 The first recordings of electrical activity of the atrioventricular bundle in humans were made by BRIAN HOFFMAN.

1959 American veterinary neuropathologist, WILLIAM HADLOW, pointed out the similarity of the brain pathology of kuru and scrapie, and the very long incubation time necessary to transmit the disease.

1959 The term 'neurolepsis' was coined by J DELAY, and J DE CASTRO, and P MUNDELEER used the term 'neurolept analgesia' in the same year.

1960   Selective uptake of norepinephrine by sympathetic nerves was demonstrated with the use of radioactive tracers by JULIUS AXELROD of the American National Institutes of Health. He discovered catechol O-methyl transferase which regulates the production of norepinephrine.

1960   The clinical effectiveness of L-dopa in patients with post-encephalitic Parkinsonism was demonstrated by British neurologist, OLIVER SACKS.

1960   A progressive neurological disorder accompanied by postural hypotension, rigidity and tremor (Shy–Drager syndrome) was described by two American neurologists, GEORGE MILTON SHY and GLEN A DRAGER.

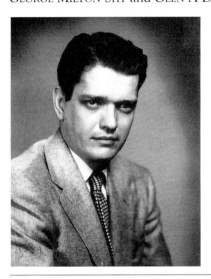

George Milton Shy
(1919–1967)

1962   Measles vaccine was developed by American bacteriologist and Nobel Prize winner, JOHN FRANKLIN ENDERS of Connecticut.

1962   BERNARD LOWEN and R AMARASINGHAM developed a direct current capacitor capable of depolarizing the myocardium transthoracically.

1963   A report was published by the Shanghai Sixth People's Hospital on the first hand transplantation, on a 27-year-old man who subsequently became a table tennis champion!

1963   A FLECKENSTEIN named calcium antagonists, a family of vasodilators which mimic the cardiac effects of calcium withdrawal.

1963   Australian neurophysiologist, SIR JOHN CAREW ECCLES, English physiologists, SIR ALAN LLOYD HODGKIN and SIR ANDREW FIELDING HUXLEY were awarded the Nobel Prize for Physiology or Medicine for their work on transmission of nerve impulses.

1964   The clinical effectiveness in patients with post-encephalitic parkinsonism of L-dopa, a current mainline drug for the treatment of Parkinson disease, was demonstrated by Viennese neurologist, O HORNYKIEWICZ.

1964   A familial disorder consisting of hyperuricemia, chorcoathetosis, mental retardation, cerebral palsy and compulsive self-mutilation (Lesch–Nyhan syndrome) was described by New York physicians, MICHAEL LESCH and WILLIAM L NYHAN.

1965   The role of acetylcholine in the transmission of nerve impulses was demonstrated by English physiologist, WILHELM SIEGMUND FELDBERG, and British pharmacologist, SIR JOHN HENRY GADDUM.

1967 Finnish-born Swedish physiologist, RAGNAR ARTHUR GRANIT, American physiologist, HALDAN KEFFER HARTLINE, and American biochemist, GEORGE WALD, were awarded the Nobel Prize for Physiology or Medicine for their work on neurophysiology of vision.

1968 A modern technique of using an open skull flap in prefrontal leucotomy was used on patients at the combined neurosurgical unit of King's College, Guy's Hospital and Maudsley Hospital.

1968 A device for delivering precise radiation to brain tumors using cobalt-60 (gamma helmet) was invented by Swedish physicists, LARS LEKSELL and BORJE LARSSON.

1968 Dizziness and the sensation of burning in the face and chest due to monosodium glutamate used in food (Chinese restaurant syndrome) was described by R H M KWOK, in the *New England Journal of Medicine*.

1968 The first prenatal diagnosis of Down syndrome through amniocentesis was made.

1969 French pediatric neurologist, JEAN AICARDI, described the combination of infantile spasms, agenesis of the corpus callosum, chorioretinal lacunae and psychomotor deterioration (Aicardi syndrome).

1970 American pharmacologist, JULIUS AXELROD, British biophysicist, SIR BERNARD KATZ, and Swedish pharmacologist, ULF SVANTE VON EULER, were awarded the Nobel Prize for Physiology or Medicine for their work on the role and mechanism of action of neurotransmitters.

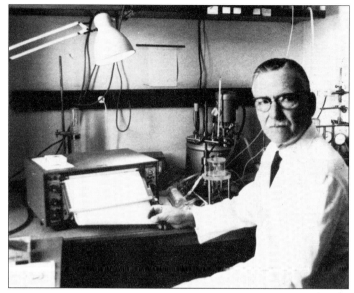

Ulf Svante von Euler (1905–1983)

1973   Computerized axial tomography (CAT) was invented by SIR
        GODFREY NEWBOLD HOUNSFIELD and ALLAN MACLEOD
        CORMACK, in England and America independently.

1973   Austrian zoologists and ethologists, KARL VON FRISCH,
        KONRAD ZACHARIAS LORENZ, and Dutch ethologist, NIKOLAAS
        TINBERGEN, were awarded the Nobel Prize for Physiology or
        Medicine for their work on animal behavior and adaptation to
        the environment.

1973   Further advances in work on enkephalins were made by
        American psychiatrist, SOLOMON HALBERT SNYDER, who
        demonstrated the presence of opiate receptors in nervous
        tissue.

1974   The first possible transmission of Creutzfeldt–Jacob disease
        from human to human was noted as the result of a corneal
        transplant.

1975   Enkephalins were identified in the treatment of pain relief by a British neurologist, HANS KOSTERLITZ.

1975   A spring-loading device for skeletal fixation of the injured spinal cord was introduced by MARIAN WEISS from Poland.

1975   ROBERT MICHAEL described the existence of calcium channels in cells.

1976   American biochemist, BARUCH SAMUEL BLUMBERG and American virologist, DANIEL CARLETON GAJDUSEK, were awarded the Nobel Prize for Physiology or Medicine for their work on hepatitis B and encephalopathy viruses.

1977   Lyme arthritis, characterized by short, recurrent attacks of asymmetric oligo-articular pain and swelling of the large joints, was reported by STEER, MALARISTA and SYNDMAN in the *American Journal of Arthritis and Rheumatism.*

1977   American pharmacologist, FERID MURAD, of Houston, analyzed how nitroglycerin and related vasodilating compounds act and discovered that they release nitric oxide which relaxes smooth muscle cells.

1977   H MOHLER and T OKADA showed that the tranquilizer, benzodiazeprine, acted on the neurotransmitter, GABA.

1977   French-born American physiologist, ROGER GUILLEMIN, Polish-born American biochemist, ANDREW VICTOR SCHALLY, and American biophysicist, ROSALYN YALOW, were awarded the Nobel Prize for Physiology or Medicine for their work on the endocrine system.

1978   The efficacy of angiotensin converting enzyme inhibitor in the treatment of congestive heart failure, was demonstrated by H GAVRAS and colleagues.

1978   The term 'toxic shock' to describe multisystem disease in seven children was first applied by J TODD and colleagues.

1979   South African-born American physicist, ALLAN MACLEOD CORMACK, and English electrical engineer, SIR GEOFFREY NEWBOLD HOUNSFIELD, were awarded the Nobel Prize for Physiology or Medicine for their development of computerized axial X-ray tomography (CAT) scanning.

1979   WHO Global Commission document signed declaring the eradication of smallpox.

1980   The Uniform Determination of Death Act was proposed by the Commission on Uniform State Laws. It stated that an individual who has sustained either irreversible cessation of circulatory and respiratory functions, or irreversible cessation of all the functions of the entire brain, including the brain stem, is dead.

1980   American pharmacologist, ROBERT F FURCHGOTT of New York, suggested that blood vessels are dilated because the endothelial cells produce an unknown signal molecule that makes vascular smooth muscle cells relax. He called this endothelium-derived relaxing factor (EDRF).

1981   Canadian-born American neurophysiologist, DAVID HUNTER HUBEL, American neuroscientist, ROGER WOLCOTT SPERRY, and Swedish neurophysiologist, TORSTEN NILS WIESEL, shared the Nobel Prize for Physiology or Medicine for their work on understanding brain nerve function and vision.

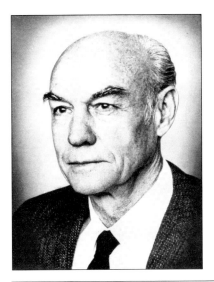

Roger Wolcott Sperry
(born 1913)

1981   The genetic code for the B surface antigen of hepatitis B was discovered in 1981, and led to the production of the first genetically engineered vaccine approved by the US Food and Drugs Administration in 1986.

1981   Uvulopalatopharyngoplasty, removal of the uvula, a portion of the soft palate and redundant tissues from the posterior wall, as treatment for obstructive sleep apnoea, was introduced by S FUJITA and coworkers.

1981   Acquired immune deficiency syndrome (AIDS) was recognized as a new disease entity, and a full description including opportunistic infections and associated neoplasms was published in the *Morbidity and Mortality Weekly Report* in June.

1982   Isolation of a new spirochete (*Borrelia burgdorferi*) from an *Ixodes* tick obtained from Staten Island, New York, by BURGDORFER. It was found to be the causative organism of Lyme disease later in the same year.

1982 An artificial heart was successfully transplanted into a human by American, Willem Kolff, keeping the patient alive for 112 hours.

1982 Stanley B Prusiner, an American neurologist in San Francisco, isolated the scrapie-causing agent, the 'prion', unlike any other known pathogen as it consists only of protein and lacks the genetic material necessary for replication.

1983 Antiphospholipid syndrome (Hughes syndrome), thrombosis, abortion and cerebral disease in the presence of lupus anticoagulant in blood, was described by G R V Hughes in the *British Medical Journal*.

1983 The gene marker for Duchenne muscular dystrophy was discovered by Kay Davies and Robert Williamson.

1983 A new retrovirus, HIV, was isolated in Paris by French molecular biologist, Luc Montagnier and colleagues at the Pasteur Institute.

1984 A transvenous catheter to deliver high-energy direct electrical current for ablation of the aberrant pathway in Wolff–Parkinson White syndrome was devised by F Morady and M M Scheinmann.

1985 The implantable defibrillator was approved by the American Food and Drug Administration.

1986 John F Kurtzke of Georgetown University School of Medicine in Washington provided evidence that multiple sclerosis was caused by a 'transmissible' agent.

1987 Implanting of cells from the adrenal gland into the brain as treatment was first proposed for treating Parkinson disease by IGNACIO NAVARRO.

1987 A protein that regulates the passage of calcium ions in and out of muscle cells during contraction and relaxation was identified by KEVIN P CAMPBELL and ROBERTO CORONADO.

1988 An attempt to apply specific criteria to, and define, 'myalgic encephalitis' (ME) was made by G P HOLMES and coworkers.

1989 The first primary myocardial disease, familial hypertrophic cardiomyopathy, to have a chromosomal locus for the defect mapped and identified was undertaken by J A JARCHO and coworkers.

1989 JOHN R. RIODAN published a paper on identification of the cystic fibrosis gene on chromosome 7.

1991 German biophysicist, ERWIN NEHER, and German electrophysiologist, BERT SAKMANN, were awarded the Nobel Prize for Physiology of Medicine for their work on electrical signals in single ion channels in membranes and development of the patch–clamp method to isolate small sections of membrane.

1992 American biochemists, EDMOND HENRI FISCHER and EDWIN GERHARD KREBS, were awarded the Nobel Prize for Physiology or Medicine for their work on the role of phosphorylation–dephosphorylation in activation of glycogen phosphorylase by adenylic acid.

1992 The transmissibility of prions to mice, rats and hamsters was demonstrated by STANLEY B PRUSINER of San Francisco.

1993 The symptoms of chronic fatigue syndrome or 'myalgic encephalitis' (ME) were shown to be due to general fatigue rather than a myalgic disorder by R H T EDWARDS and colleagues.

1994 American pharmacologist, ALFRED GOODMAN GILMAN, shared the Nobel Prize for Physiology or Medicine with American biochemist, MARTIN RODBELL, for their work on G proteins, intermediates in the pathway of cells in response to incoming signals.

1996 SHINGO MURAKAMI, a Japanese virologist, found traces of the herpes simplex virus in facial nerves of patients with Bell palsy.

1996 American neurologist, STANLEY PRUSINER'S work on the prion received acceptance with the recognition of new variant Creutzfeldt–Jakob disease in Britain.

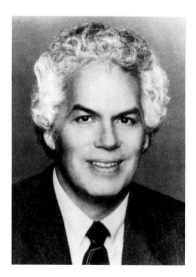

Stanley Prusiner
(born 1942)

1997   American neurologist and biochemist, STANLEY PRUSINER, received the Nobel Prize for his discovery of the prion as an infectious protein, lacking nucleic acid, and causing transmissible spongiform encephalopathies.

1998   The Nobel Prize in Physiology or Medicine was jointly awarded to American scientists, ROBERT F FURCHGOTT of New York, LOUIS J IGNARRO and FERID MURAD of Los Angeles for their discoveries concerning nitric oxide as a signaling molecule in the cardiovascular system.

1998   CARL HELLERQVIST and colleagues at the Vanderbilt University in Nashville showed that giving an experimental drug consisting of a polysaccharide from streptococci can block spinal cord injury in mice, allowing growth of new blood vessels.

1999   ZEMPHIRA ALAVIDZE and colleagues of the University of Maryland School of Medicine have found a way of using bacteriophages to infect and kill *Pseudomonas aeruginosa*, a bacterium responsible for most deaths of cystic fibrosis patients.

1999   KARIN NELSON of the National Institutes of Health, and JUDITH GRETHER of the California Birth Defects Monitoring Program suggested that inflammation during pregnancy, rather than lack of oxygen, can cause cerebral palsy in the newborn.

1999   GÜNTER BLOBEL of the Rockefeller University in New York was awarded the Nobel Prize for Physiology or Medicine for his discovery that proteins have intrinsic signals that govern their transport and localization in the cell. This research aids understanding of the molecular mechanisms involved in many genetic diseases, such as cystic fibrosis or hyperoxaluria, and of the functioning of the immune system.